BE ALIVE

A N D

CANCER FREE

Dr. Gabriel O. Nnanna

Reviewed by:

DR. HENRY N. CHINEKE
Senior Lecturer/ Consultant Family Medicine

CMAC IMSUTH, ORLU, NIGERIA.

ISBN: 9798851159794

Printed in Nigeria by Rex Press
Christ The King Cathedral
P.M.B. 7526, Aba, Abia State – Nigeria
October 2016

DEDICATION

To my bosom friend professor Okey Okorafor who has fought his metastatic liver cancer for 2 years but succumbed finally.

 To the chronically ill cancer patients who, out of poverty and ignorance, suffer and die in most undignified manners.
To my lecturers and Batch 3 DFM students of the National Post Graduate Medical College of Nigeria (NPMCN), Awka study center, who have made me understand that updating medical knowledge has no age limit but rather most rewarding in our medical practice.

To my late brother Chief Vincent O. Nnanna who toiled at the end of the Nigerian civil war to make me attain my present educational status as a medical Doctor.

ACKNOWLEDEMENT

I am very grateful to the Almighty God who made it possible that I be alive to produce the second edition of BE ALIVE AND CANCER FREE.

The interest shown by many people today in diet and physical activities as means of healthy leaving is demonstrated by the number of congratulatory messages that keep flooding my mail box. I am glad you are thinking that way now.

The demonstration by Dr. Lorraine Day, Professor Jane Plant and Dr. Batmanghelidj that we can ameliorate or even cure cancers through what we eat still burns in me. I continue to be grateful to them for leading me into the secrets of healthy living in our diets.

I will live to remember Dr. A.E.Tetenta, N. Eleweke, J. Ojiabo C. K. Chima and Professor R.U. Ononogbo who stood by me when I had prostate cancer.

I remain grateful to Evangelist Dr. H. N. Chineke, Chairman Medical Advisory Committee, IMSUTH, Orlu, for the great interest he showed in reviewing this book. The forward for this edition which he wrote, is a testimony that he read every word of this book. He also made a lot of contributions to give the book its present high quality.

I cannot forget my wife and children who stood by me during the production of this work. My daughter Mabel, I owe you so much for typing the whole book. My other children – Oleka, Anthony and Emeka were always on the phone to encourage me. I thank you all.

I appreciate the comments of many whom I cannot mention that sent me greetings on the first edition and wish all will benefit from the contents of this edition.

May God bless you all who will find this book useful in changing their diets and life style.

Dr. G. O. Nnanna

FOREWARD

Many publications, treatise, abstracts and books have been published on health and human nutrition, but this very one by my erudite scholar and colleague, Dr. Gabriel O. Nnanna is a real classique!. You are what you eat. Many people dig their graves with their teeth as a result of improper nutrition, Often caused by ignorance and not necessarily financial lack. This negative health complication culminate in increased morbidity, mortality and the overall reduction of the human life span.

As a specialist, involved the practice of family medicine daily, I wished to unequivocally state that majority of human ailments can be remotely traced to a nutritional problem. This masterpiece therefore is a worthy contribution by Dr. Nnanna geared towards preventing and ameliorating the declining state of health of our people, and we are indeed grateful.

I strongly recommend this book to all viz: families, secondary and post-secondary school students, traders, business men, the clergy, women groups, hotels and hospitality outfits, eateries, dieticians, family physicians as well as those involved in researches related to food, nutrition and health.

Dr. Henry Nnaemeka Chineke

AUTHOR'S NOTE

The information contained in this book were based on works by many researchers. Notable among them were Dr. L. Day and Dr. F. Batmanghelidj. Other information were gathered from summaries of natural healing plants edited by Mr. Chukwuma Muanya of the Nigerian Guardian Newspapers. My personal experiences in the last eight years have been very rewarding. I feel I should share the knowledge with those who do not have the opportunities that have come my way.

However, the contents of this book do not intend to make you your personal doctor. Your medical doctor is indispensable at all times as the information contained here should not replace treatments from your medical doctor. To do otherwise is at your own risk, as neither I, the author, nor my agents will be held liable. It is however, advisable to draw my attention to the information contained herein if you so desire.

I have tried to avoid the use of medical terminologies to enable every reader understand fully the contents of this book. Where these terms are un-avoidable, attempts are made to explain them. There are repetitions at several areas of the book. They are deliberate and meant for emphasis.

Since knowledge is dynamic, more information which have emerged since the 1st edition in 2011 and comments from our readers have necessitated the review of some parts of this book.

Dr. G.O. Nnanna

CONTENTS   Pages

CHAPTER ONE

INTRODUCTION

Diseases that afflict us are results of the interactions between our internal and external environments. The worst culprits here are stress, toxins in the air, water, diet and those produced by the body and microorganisms in foods and air. Even when people live in the same community many do not suffer the prevalent diseases because of their internal environments, which are controlled by their life styles and genetic makeups. Our life styles directly determine the ability of our immune system to withstand and protect us against diseases including cancers.

WHAT IS CANCER

DEFINITION

Tumour: this is a mass of cells growing abnormally where they should not, causing medical problems.

Tumours may be

(a) Benign or non-malignant tumour: This grows slowly only at one part of the body and not likely to cause death of the patient or spread to other parts of the body.

Examples: Lipomas, fibroids and benign prostatic hyperplasia (BPH--enlargement)

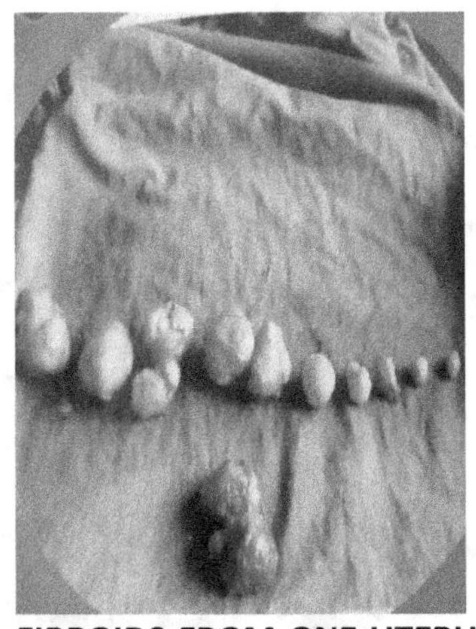

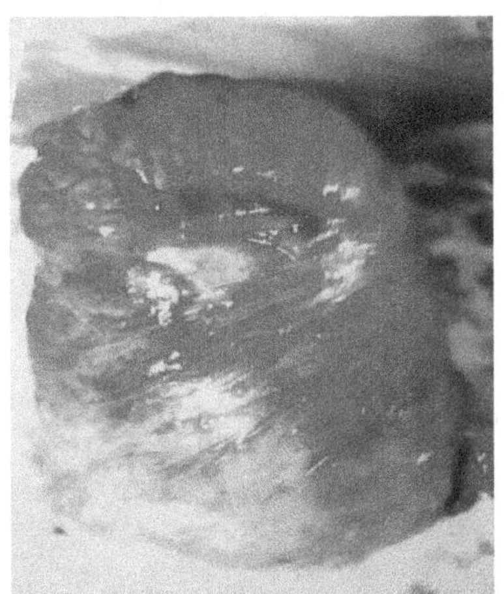

FIBROIDS FROM ONE UTERUS
HYPERPLESIA

BENIGN   PROSTATIC

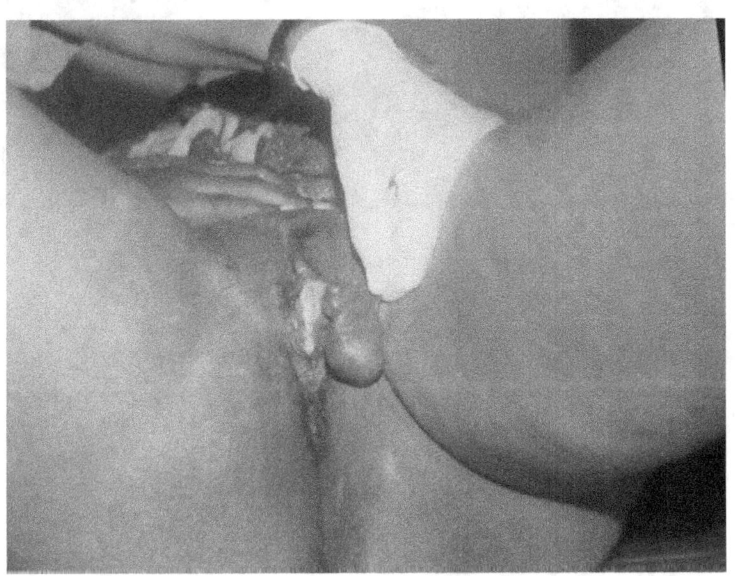

BENIGN GROWTH AFTER FEMALE GENITAL MUTILATION
(SEBACEOUS CYST)

(b) **Malignant tumour or cancer. The tumour grows faster. Its growth cannot be controlled and is likely to cause death. It can invade other parts of the body. Examples: prostate cancer, cervical and breast cancers.**

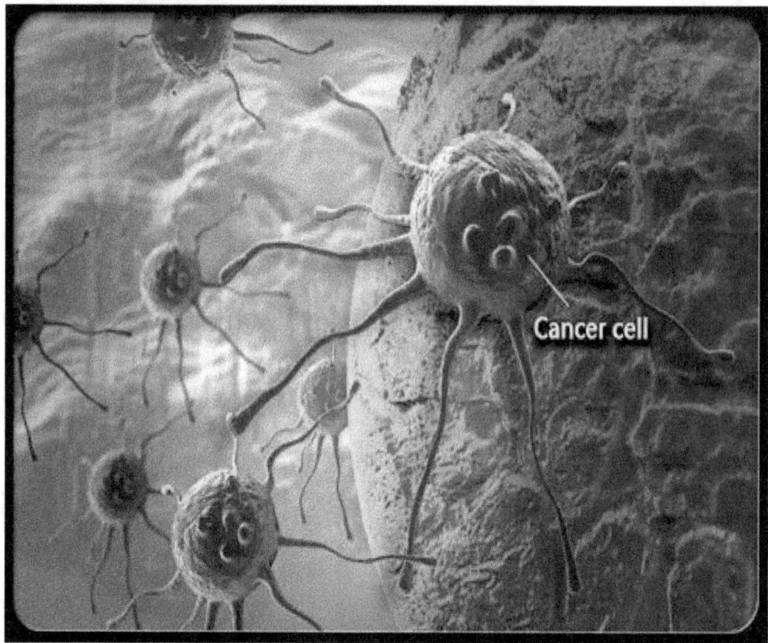

TYPICAL CANCER CELL

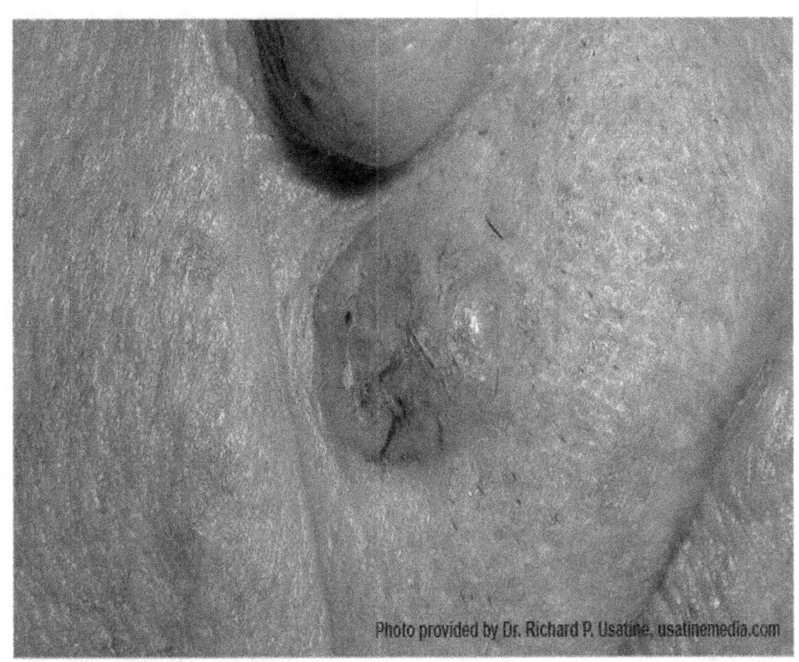

SKIN CANCER (MELANOMA)

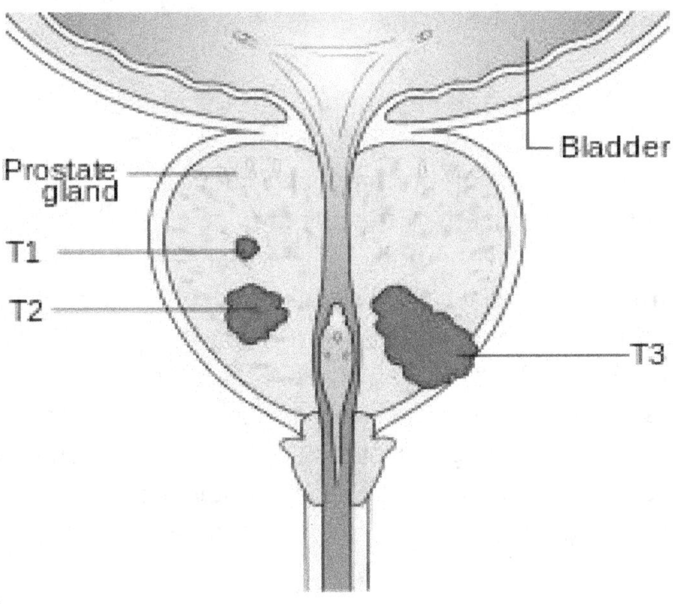

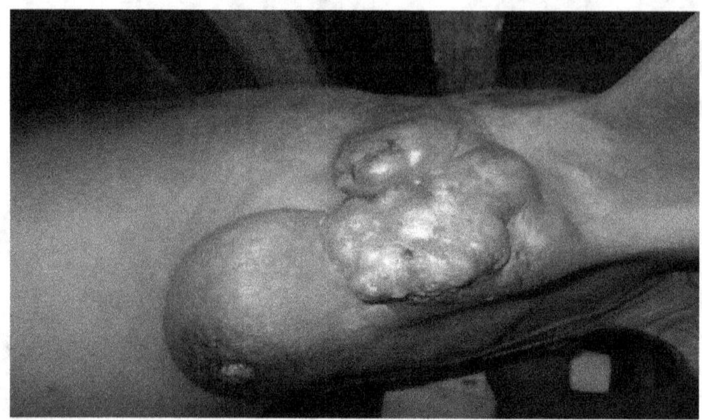

BREAST CANCER

CHARACTERISTICS OF CANCER CELLS
They are primitive and genetically selfish
They thrive in low oxygen (anaerobic) conditions
They exhibit stem cell characteristics as they try to differentiate into new organs which they invade.

(1)   The cells break natural boundaries of mother organs and spread (metastasis) rapidly to invade other organs resulting in fatal disruptions of normal body functions to the point of exhaustion and death of their victims.

As cells of the body mature they develop sophisticated communication skills. These skills control growth of individual cells and organ boundaries.

By this 'social sophistication' the cells of the body respect one another and are not selfish. Cancer cells have lost this social skills, subsequently grow into masses that break boundaries and encroach on spaces allocated to their neighbours and even away from their primary point of origin (metastasis).

(2)The cancer cells live and thrive in low oxygen and very acidic environments where normal cells will not. Normal cells perform optimally in alkaline environments PH 7.2 – 7.4. Chlorophylls, vegetables and fruits contribute a lot to the alkaline nature of the body fluids.

(3)They have capabilities to achieve sophistication and develop very poor characteristics of other cells in the organs they invade, displacing the cells of the organ yet are not able to perform the full functions of these organs. This results to the poor health conditions of their victims.

(4) Cancer cells reproduce so rapidly that they do not have time to differentiate and mature.

(5) Normal cells can repair themselves if their genes become damaged or die (apoptosis) but cancer cells do not repair themselves.

(6) The activities of these cancer cells suppress the immune system and subsequently overwhelm the body. This result in the deplorable condition we find our cancer patients.

FORMATION OF CANCER CELLS

All cancers begin with changes (mutations) in one of the 100 billion cells of the body.

The interior of normal cells maintain an alkaline state of about PH 7.4. In dehydration (low water content) the intracellular fluid becomes acidic. Together with toxin (poisons) and OXYRADICALS, the internal environments are altered. The free radicals can cause the DNA to fuse with other proteins inside the cells through a process known as cross – linking. This can result to alteration of delicate structures of the cells including the DEOXYRIBONUCEIC ACID (DNA). Mutation may occur. The DNAs in normal cells are repaired if the cells are adequately rehydrated and toxins removed. When DNA damages outstrip repair, mutations persist. These altered DNAs replicate to produce cancer cells.

CANCER STAGING

Some Clinicians use the staging system called the TNM (Tumour Node Metastasis) system for most cancers. Based on the TNM system, cancer staging is as follows:

STAGE 0: This is cancer in situ, which means the cancer is in its place of origin.

STAGE 1: The cancer is relatively small and contained within the organ. Early stage cancer penetrates beyond original layer of tissue.

STAGE 2: The cancer is larger than in stage 1 and have spread to the lymph nodes close to the cancer.

STAGE 3: The cancer is larger. It has started spreading into surrounding tissues plus cancer cells in the lymph nodes.

STAGE 4: The cancer has spread from where it started to other body organs. This is called the secondary or metastatic cancer.

Cancer severity is divided into four stages (as above) with severity increasing from I to IV. Stages I & II have good survival rates. These are stages where conventional treatments make a difference for some cancer patients at great sacrifices for the patients and families who live with serious side effects and financial burdens. Today, survival rates among these two stages have markedly improved especially in the developed countries due to great advances in Medicare in those countries. In stage IV surgery, chemotherapy or radiation generally do not work with regard to prolongation of life, but rather makes lives of patients and relations more difficult.

No organ of the body is spared by cancers, however, cancers are divided into the following types.

CANCER TYPES	EXAMPLES
Carcinoma	Malignancy of epithelial cell of organs; Skin, large intestines, Bronchi, Prostate, Breast ,Cervix and Stomach
Sarcomas	Malignancy of mesodermal cells origin as connective tissues--- Cartilages, striated muscles, Bone marrow and other blood forming organs which produce abnormal immature leucocytes and suppress formation of other blood cells.
Lymphomas	Malignancy of lymphoid organs, Non Hodgkin Lymphoma(Burkitt's), Hodgkin Lymphomas
Leukaemia	Malignancy of white blood cells
Brain Tumours	Abnormal cell growth in the brain

FACTORS THAT CONTRIBUTE TO CANCER FORMATION/RISKS FACTORS

AGE: cancer most commonly develop in older people.78% of all cancers are diagnosed in people 55years and above. However people who smoke, eat unhealthy diet or are physically inactive have a higher risks of cancers for their ages.

GENETIC INHERITANCE: Cancers found in families are traced to their genetic make ups (Genes/DNAs).

Some of these include:

(a) Breast and ovarian cancers.

(b) Colon (large intestine) and endometrial (uterus) cancers

(c) Colo-rectal cancers

EXTERNAL ENVIRONMENTS

Polluted environments from automobile exhaust fumes (carbon monoxide)

Tobacco which causes lung, bladder, head and neck cancers.

Alcohol which causes oesophageal (gullet) and liver cancers.

Aflatoxin: Toxin from fungi (aspergillus) infested food causes liver cancer. It is one of the most potent non carcinogens known to mankind.

Occupation: Inhalation of chemicals and asbestos in factories cause lung cancers and chronic obstructive pulmonary disease (COPD).

Ultra-violet (UV) from sunlight.

It causes skin cancers especially in albinos.

THE INTERNAL ENVIRONMENTS

The production of oxy-radicals from body metabolism and dehydration (as mentioned above).

Nutrition: Recent studies have shown that nutrition and lifestyle affect significantly the expression of genes in diseases. Example, active lifestyle can reduce breast cancer risk by 50% compared to sedentary lifestyle.

Western diet, plenty meat, fatty foods, empty calories from fast (dead) foods and beverages contribute markedly to increase incidents of cancer. Examples: colorectal and breast cancers.

GEOGRAPHICAL DISTRIBUTION OF CANCERS

Cancers are found all over the world in every organ of the body but the incidence and type may differ from one geographical region to another.

The commonest cancers world-wide include

Breast

Prostate

Cervix

Lungs

Bladder

Ovarian

Non Hodgkin lymphomas, (Burkitt's)

Hodgkin's lymphoma

Leukaemia and

 Ano-rectal cancers

Pancreatic cancer though rare is very aggressive with very poor survival rates worldwide, of less than 5%.

CANCERS WITH POTENTIALS FOR SCREENING

S/N	Malignancy/cancer	Method
1	Breast cancer	Mammography
2	Cervical cancer	Cervical smear cytology

3	Prostate cancer	Prostate specific antigen (PSA), 4 quadrant biopsy, Trans - Rectal ultra sound
4	Colorectal cancer	Simple sigmoidoscopy and faecal occult blood test

Since these cancers have potentials for screening, they can therefore be detected at stages 0 to 2 when survival rates are still very high.

SOME VITAL CANCER AND NON COMMUNICABLE DISEASE (NCD) STATISTICS

Chronic non-communicable diseases including cancers, kill nearly 35 million people per year. Almost 90 percent of fatalities before the age of 60 occur in developing world and are largely preventable. In developing countries, the communicable diseases are more in the rural areas but the non-communicable diseases (NCDs) are more in the urban centres because these are diseases of lifestyle, e.g. smoking, alcohol, sedentary lifestyles and affluence. A recent U.K. studies (Lancet, N=1million) has shown that about 6 million people die of smoking each year. Sedentary office work of up to 8hours a day is cause of sudden death of 5.3 million people each year. "The NCDs are one of the world's fastest growing and most alarming health problems" (Dr. M. Cham; D.G. WHO. 63rd All World Health Assembly 2010). Heart diseases are still a major killer in the entire world. Worldwide, heart attacks and stroke account for 25 percent of deaths per annum.

Death profiles of few recent years:

Projected main causes of death worldwide, all ages.
2005. Total deaths: 59 million.
Cardiovascular disease/stroke: 17.5 million.

- Cancer: 7.5 million. Or 13%
- Chronic respiratory disease: 4.2 million.
- Diabetes 1.16 million.
- Other chronic diseases 5.2 million.

In 2012, of the 14 million cases of cancer diagnosed, 8.2million died worldwide (world cancer research fund international report 2012)

Some estimated number of new cancer cases and deaths by sex: US 2015 for all types of cancer.

	Site /Organ	NEW CASES			ESTIMATED DEATHS		
		Both Sexes	Male	Female	Both sexes	Male	Female
1	All sites	1,658,370	848,200	810,170	589,430	312,150	227,280
2	Colon	93,090	45,890	47,200	49,700	26,100	23,600
3	Rectum	39,610	23,200	16,410	-	-	-
4	Pancreas	48,960	24,840	24,120	40,560	20,710	19,850
5	Lungs & Bronchus	221,200	115,610	105,590	158,040	86,380	71,600
6	Breast	234,190	2,350	231,840	40,730	44	40,290
7	Uterine Cervix	12,900	-	12,900	4,100	-	4,100
8	Uterine Corpus (body)	54,870	-	54,870	10,170	-	10,170
9	Prostrate	220,800	220,800	-	27,540	27,540	-
10	Non Hodgkin lymphoma (NHL)	71,850	39,850	32,000	19,790	11,480	8,310
11	Hodgkin lymphoma	9,050	5,100	3,950	1,150	660	490
12	Leukemia	54,270	30,900	23,370	24,450	14,210	10,240

Source: 1995-2011 incidence rates reported by North American Association of Central Cancers Registries (NAACCR)

These data show that 36% of American cancer patients died in 2015; 454.5/day and 189/hr or 3/min. What could be the situation in Nigeria where national statistics are not available and coupled with the poor level of our health facilities.

UK CANCER STATISTICS

Total 2014 UK-352,129 total new cases 161,823 deaths. This translates to 46% of British cancer patients died in 2014; 443.4 deaths in 1 day or 18.5 deaths/hour.

Breast Cancer 2012: deaths; 11,600 women died from breast cancer which is about 32 everyday

About 75 men died from breast cancer in UK

2012 – 1,200 deaths from breast cancer in women < 50 years.

In UK 2012 breast cancer was second most common cancer in women after lung cancer.

It is estimated that worldwide 522,000 women died of breast cancer in 2012 with varying rates across the world.

Prostate cancer

47,300 new cases in 2013

10,837 deaths in 2012

Lung cancer

45,525 new cases in 2013,

35,375 deaths in 2012

This cancer is 95% preventable without smoking

Bowel cancer

41,112 new cases in 2013

16,187 deaths in 2012

57% have survival rate of 10 or more years.

(From cancer Research UK 2013)

NIGERIA CANCER STATISTICS/SITUATION

The burden of cancer in Nigeria is unknown because of lack of statistics or under-reporting as in most African countries. It is among 3rd leading causes of death in developing countries (Fatima Abdul Kareem. LUTH)

There are 11 cancer registries in Nigeria, and except that at UCH, are properly funded. Only few hospital based data are available. Similar to studies from developed countries, cancer is slightly higher in female than men in Nigeria.

6 Most common cancers in Nigeria in decreasing order of frequency are

breast- peak 5th decade

Cervical – between 17-80years

Prostrate - >10times more in African Americans men aged 60.5 – 71.4 years

Colorectal – accounts for 10 – 50% of GIT cancers in Nigeria. Incidence is increasing because fibre diet is substituted with highly refined foods. Cancer age is 60 – 70 years

Liver: Most common cancer cause of deaths in Nigeria

NHL (Non-Hodgkin's Lymphoma)

Breast cancers occur more in menopausal women with peak age of 5th decade. Male breast cancer represents 3.7 – 8.86% of all breast cancers, higher than other parts of the world.

The World Health Organization (WHO, 2008) has warned on the rise of cancer cases in developing countries, which account for 70 percent of all cancer deaths and 63 percent of new cases. In 2004, 7.4 million cancer deaths occurred globally, 63 percent in developing countries. In 2008, 12.7 million new cases and 7.6 million cancer deaths occurred globally; this could rise to 13 million in 2030. 100,000 cancer deaths occur in Nigeria yearly (Fed. Min. of Health 2009)

Nigeria has the highest cancer deaths in Africa (WHO 2013). 250,000 cases are recorded annually. Only 17% of African countries are sufficiently funding cancer controlled programs. In Nigeria, many still see cancer as disease of the wealthy, elderly and of developed countries"therefore it is their business".

Globally, cervical cancer claims the life of a woman every two minutes. 8,000 women will die of cervical cancer every year in painful, miserable and undignified manners in Nigeria. 80 percent of affected women in Nigeria present themselves in very advanced stages III & IV when very little may be done to prolong their lives.

In Sub-Saharan Africa, a woman dies every 10 minutes from cervical cancer. In Nigeria, cervical cancer is second to breast cancer in women in the south but is the first in the north, based on data from our teaching hospitals. 80 percent of cervical cancer patients in Africa will die of the disease while in Asia it is 50 percent and less than 50 percent in Europe and North America. (FMOH 2009)

Cervical cancer is caused by the human papilloma virus (HPV) which is a sexually transmitted disease linked to 97.7 percent of cases. Screening program for HPV is now available for early detection, treatment and prevention before it progresses to full blown cancer.

No fewer than 3 million Nigerians are living with cancer.
Over 100,000 others are queuing to enlist yearly.
This could rise to 500,000 by 2020 if nothing drastic is

done now to avert the situation. (FMOH 2010 Guardian 11/02/10)

7,000-10,000 new cases of breast cancer are recorded in Nigeria yearly (Nigeria Guardian 04/02/10.) Most African cases are diagnosed in 10- 15 years (younger) women than in developed countries. At the Lagos University Teaching Hospitals (LUTH), out of every 10 cancer cases, 5 are breast cancer, 3 are cervical, while 2 are other types of cancer (Anozie E. Guardian 11/02/10) Cancer in women in Nigeria fuels poverty since it affects mostly the poorest women who are both providers and care givers.

Prostate, Liver and lung cancers are common in   men,   with prostate cancer as the predominant   one.

WHO estimates that 84 million people will die of cancer between 2005 and 2015 without intervention

Commonest cancers in Nigeria are

Breast

Cervix

Prostrate

Colorectal

Liver

Non-Hodgkin's Lymphoma

Significant numbers of breast cancer are also seen in men (Fatima Abdul Kareem-LUTH)

Factors responsible for increasing incidence (Risk factors) of cancer and other non-communicable diseases (NCDs) in Nigeria and other developing countries include:

Aging population. Higher life expectancy is also associated with cancers, 78% of cancers occur in 55years and above

Low medical awareness of prevention and early detection of cancers.

Little or no access to diagnostic facilities.

Non-Empowerment of women to make independent decisions about their health care.
Smoking.
Increasing change to Western diet.
Physical inactivity and obesity.
Obstetrics and Gynecological factors.
Oncology centers in Nigeria are ill equipped

Recent studies also blame:
1.	Air Pollution especially traffic pollution which fosters diabetes, breast cancer and chronic lung 		disease (Env. HL perspectives)
2.	Heavy metal contamination of underground waters from wells, boreholes and shallow streams.
3.	Radiation from high tension electric lines.
4.	Cell phones.
It is unfortunate critics may say "the future is bleak in Nigeria":

1.	With no solid National cancer control programs.
2.	Apparent lack of accessibility of cancer diagnosis and treatment
3.	Non availability and non-affordability of treatment modalities.
4.	Low capacity for cancer management.
5.	With the country's precarious health indices "Cancer will continue to have a field day" upon the 		.		hapless populace in the developing countries, and Nigeria in particular.

For the way forward experts agree on the following:

1.	Early detection through regular screening.
2.	Lifestyle changes
Water therapy

Not smoking

Moderate or no-alcohol

Eating plant-based and traditional foods

3.   Re-equipping tertiary hospitals with state-of-the-art equipment-CT scan, mammographic scan,   .   Magnetic Resonance Imaging (MRI) machines to detect cancers.

4.   Specialized cancer training for all medical workers.

5.   Hospitals to care for terminally ill patients.

6.   Comprehensive health education programs at all levels of education.

7.   HPV detection procedures at health centers and general hospitals.

8.   Train more oncologists to handle cancer cases.

Clinical services for cancer are grossly inadequate and poorly distributed. Only few functional radiotherapy equipment are available, where access is limited by costs.

Chemotherapy and pathology services are available but high costs prevent most patients from accessing them.

Cancer surgeries are performed by surgeons not specialized in oncology.

Since most patients present with advanced diseases, treatments that offer prospects of prolonged survival are limited. Though most federal Government Teaching Hospitals have oncology units, services offered are limited. The only option left for rich Nigerians is to travel abroad for better management that can add years to their lives.

Today conventional orthodox treatments for cancers that show great prospects include:

1.	Surgery for removal of part or whole of the affected organ-excision biopsy
2.	Hormone therapy
3	Immune therapy
4.	Targeted therapy, drugs that specifically interfere with cancer cell growth. This is possible through the Human Genome Project (HGP).This project which lasted 13 years was completed in 2004. It has opened a very wide door for medicine and biotechnology developments.

The severe side effects of each of these treatments above are well known to every Clinician, especially the oncologists (Cancer specialist). Some of these side effects include:
1.	Depression of the immune (defense) system resulting in high susceptibility of the individuals to infections, as seen with chemotherapy and radiotherapy. The patient becomes very weak because of the depressed immune system.

2.	Increased fragility of bones due to radiations resulting in frequent fractures that hardly heal. It is common knowledge that radiographers, taking radiographs, in a routine investigation like chest X-ray wear shields and stand behind lead walls to prevent exposure to the x-rays. But this is the standard treatment for Cancers. Cancers are not caused by x-ray deficiencies. While radiating the cancer cells the normal cells are not spared, resulting in necrosis and fistulae (channels between two surfaces) as in prostate cancer radiations. However, this treatment is of great value for stages I & II

3.	Surgery results in direct metastasis (spread) of the cancer cells to other vital organs, like the liver. Lymph nodes, the store houses of defense, white blood cells including Natural Killers (N.K) cells in lymph nodes are removed, thus rendering the defense system ineffective. It should be noted that excision biopsy could add more years to the life of stages I & II cancer patients.

Today, there are remedies that are not causing hair loss, bone marrow depression, not destroying the immune system or causing faecal or urinary incontinence. There are natural treatments for breast and prostate cancers that prove to be very effective and successful.

THE NEW PARADIGM

Today, the attitude of taking care of the body when we are ill is giving way to the realization that it is preferable to prevent a health problem to treating it. The improved life expectancy in developed countries is due to a shift in two directions: On the one hand due to advances in medical technology and on the other, due to interest in complementary and alternative medicine (CAM) which focuses on fitness, lifestyles, diet, emotional, spiritual health and physical exercises. Early detection of diseases including NCDs and cancer is another area we are lagging behind the developed countries. This is why many orthodox medical practitioners are crossing the great divide to complementary and alternative medicines. This results to a shift towards more comprehensive therapies for the whole person. This is the holistic bio –psychosocial model of health care which is patient centered medicine.(Engel 1977) Physicians should explore presenting complaints and hidden actual reasons for coming (ARC) to the physician. This falls within the domain of the family physician.   In 2002, 36 percent of USA citizens used complementary and alternative medicine at any time. It was 62 percent if prayers for health were added. Today many are opting for CAM because of lack of confidence in conventional medicines because of their side effects, costs and lack of state of the art medical equipment for diagnosis and treatment in the developing countries. (See conclusion). On the other hand CAM is considered as very safe. In 1998 drugs side effect was the sixth most common cause of death, in USA (Washington post 15/04/98).

The fact that people in the developing countries cannot afford regular medical checks as in developed countries, results in diagnosis of our diseases at very late stages. This is because so many personal, family and community needs are competing for the meager financial resources available to us. Doctors are now emphasizing on diet, lifestyles changes, physical exercise and spiritual wellbeing as integral components of health maintenance and therapy through balanced diet, fresh natural foods, regulated dietary regimens, vitamin supplements, regular medical checks, and other natural products. The common cancers occur as a result of the environments; internal and external in which we live and are therefore, in principle, preventable and curable. There are very strong evidences that most of the cancers could be made less severe and cured by modifications of our lifestyles and regular medical checks.

RREVENTION OF CANCERS
A substantial proportion of cancers could be prevented or their effects minimized.
All cancers caused by tobacco use and heavy alcohol consumption could be prevented. In 2015 almost 171,000 of the estimated 589,430 cancer deaths in USA were caused by tobacco smoking.
 One third of US cancers are related to overweight or obesity, physical inactivity and or processed foods and thus could be prevented.
Certain cancers are related to infective agents
Human Papilloma Virus (HPV) for cervical cancers.
Hepatitis B virus (HBV) and hepatitis C virus (HCV)
both for liver cancers
Human Immune Deficiency virus (HIV) for skin cancers.
Helicobacter pylori (H. pylori) for stomach cancers.
These cancers can be prevented by either
Behavioral changes
Vaccinations or
Treating the infections responsible

The more than 3 million skin cancers diagnosed annually can be prevented by protecting the skin from excessive sun exposure.
Screening can prevent colorectal, prostate and cervical cancers by early detection and removal of pre-cancerous lesions.
Breast cancer can be prevented by personal examination of the breast while mammography can detect cancer "in-situ" or stage 1 cancer which can then be excised.

THE IMMUNE SYSTEM

Further discussions will dwell on how the immune system, our lifestyles and diets can be means of achieving good health and cure of chronic diseases and cancers.
We are ill when our immunity to diseases breaks down. This is as a result of our genetics, improper diets and habits which produce toxins and oxy - radicals which affect the body at the cellular level. When we are ill we expect our doctors to cure us but fail to realize that "The Cure" comes from within -the wondrous immune system. If we boost our immune system, our diseases especially the chronic diseases and cancers can be prevented or cured. The inescapable stress of our life-style predisposes us to:
1.   Cancers,
2.   Cardiovascular diseases like heart attacks, stroke, hypertension,
3.   Viral disorders; common cold and herpes, AIDS and hepatitis B&C. There is hardly any disease that stress does not play an aggravating role or any part of the body that is not affected by it.
 The immune system is our personal security / defense guard. Because of the importance of this system to further discussions in this book, we shall explore it more with a view to appreciate it.

The immune system consists of a network of cells, proteins and lymphoid organs located in different parts of the body intricately linked by lymph vessels. The system ensures maximum protection against external and internal foreign bodies, which try to upset the balanced functions of different parts of the body (Davidson's Principles and Practice of Medicine 20th Edition). Immune Responses may be

(1)   Innate / Immediate - Which provides immediate reaction to protect the body and

(2)   Adaptive or Acquired or Delayed Response: This takes longer time to develop but are specific and offer longer lasting protection.

PROPERTIES OF IMMUNE RESPONSES

Innate	Adaptive/Delayed
	Characteristics
(1) Recognizes genetically microbial Structures.	Antigen specific Responses.

(2)	Mobilized within minutes	Slow response (days)
(3)	No memory	has memory
(4)	Genetically encoded (Inherent)	not genetically coded
(5)	Identical responses in all Individuals'	Acquired as adaptive response to Exposures to antigens

IMMUNE	**COMPONENTS**
(1) Constitutive barriers e.g. Skin	(1) T and B lymphocytes
(2) Phagocytes	(2) Secreted molecules - Antibodies
(3) Natural killers (T - Cells)	(3) Antigen specific receptors
(4) Cytotoxic T - cells	
(5) Complements	
(6) Cytokines	
(7) Helper T - cells	

(Adapted from Davidson's principles of medicine 20th edition p65).

THE INNATE IMMUNE SYSTEM CONSIST OF:

(1) Phagocytes (eating cells): These are specialized cells.

Functions:
(1) Ingest and kill micro - organisms
(2) Scavenge cellular and infectious debris
(3) Produce inflammatory molecules that influence other components of the immune system.

Phagocytes Include
Neutrophils
Monocytes
Macrophages
These are very important for defense against bacterial and fungal infections.

(2)   CYTOKINES: They are small soluble proteins that act as multi - purpose chemical messengers

Some important Cytokines in the immune system include:

(1)   Interferon alpha - Produced by T - cells, NK cells and macrophages. Interferon has antiviral
        activities. It activates NK cells and macrophages and C D8 T cells.
(2)   Interferon gamma - Produced by T cells. It increases antimicrobial and anti-tumor activities of   Macrophages.

(3)   Tumor necrosis factor alpha - Produced by macrophages increases apoptosis (gradual cell
death). They are directly cytotoxic.

(4)   Interleukins are produced by macrophages, monocytes and   neutrophils.   They   stimulate
        maturation of B & T cells; production of antibodies and maturation of B - Cells into plasma cells.

(5)   Complements: They are a group of over 20 proteins that promote inflammation and eliminate   Invading pathogens by osmotic cell lysis. (Rupture of cell walls with content escape)

(6)   CYTOTOXIC T - CELLS: They destroy cancerous cells, viruses inflected   cells and allografts (living   tissue taken from one person to another: transplanted). Their actions are selectively specific.

(7)   NULL CELLS: These are a small proportion of lymphoid cells, which originate in the bone   marrow, but are neither T nor B lymphocytes. Some are KILLER (K) cells with cytotoxic properties   against target cells coated with antibodies. Others are Natural Killers (N.K) cells which have lytic   functions against certain tumour cells and virally infected   cells.

(8)   Helper T Cells: Stimulate production of cytotoxic cells which destroy antigen presenting cells and cancerous cells.

ADAPTIVE / ACQUIRED IMMUNE SYSTEM
The two arms of adaptive immune responses are:-
(1)   Humoral Immunity - mediated by antibodies produced
        by B lymphocytes.
(2)   Cellular Immune Responses - Mediated by T lymphocytes which synthesize and release cytokines. Both innate and adaptive immune systems work closely to maximize the effectiveness of the immune system.

LYMPHOID ORGANS.
These are organs responsible for production of lymphocytes
(1)   Primary lymphoid organs are involved in production of lymphocytes. They include bone marrow where   both T and B lymphocytes are produced. B lymphocytes mature in the bone marrow, while T lymphocytes mature in the thymus.

(2) Secondary lymphoid organs: After maturation, Lymphocytes migrate to the secondary lymphoid organs. These include (1)

lymph nodes (2) Mucosa Associated Lymph Tissues (MALT). These organs trap and concentrate foreign substances and tumor cells. They are the major sites of interaction between lymphocytes and microorganisms and   tumor cells. MALT Consists of

(a)   lymphoid cells in gut (Payer's patches and Lamina propria).

(b)   In the pharynx are tonsils and adenoids and

(c)   Sub-mucosal lymphoid tissues (Waldeyer's ring).

(3)   Spleen: It's a major site of antibody synthesis and filters the blood.

(4)   Lymph nodes: They maximize drainage of lymph from different parts of the body.

The lymphocytes (lymph vessels): The lymphocytes connect the lymphoid tissues.

(1)   They provide access to lymph nodes- afferent and efferent vessels.

(2)   Return tissue fluid from interstitial spaces to the venous system.

(3)   Transport fat from small intestine into blood stream.

They begin as extracellular interstitial spaces which coalesce to form the ducts which enter and leave the lymph nodes as afferent and efferent ducts. The ducts coalesce to drain into thoracic duct and subsequently into the superior vena cava.

HUMORAL IMMUNITY

B lymphocytes

Their main function is to produce antibodies. They encounter foreign bodies in the lymph nodes where they are provided with appropriate signals from T-Lymphocytes to proliferate by a process known as "clonal Expansion". Further differentiations produce either long lived memory cells which reside in the lymph nodes or plasma cells which produce antibodies.

Immunoglobulin (Antibodies): They facilitate
(1)   Phagocytosis by acting as opsonins (which make bacteria more attractive for   phagocytosis)
(2)   Cell killing by cytotoxic cells especially NK cells.
(3)   Antibody-   Antigen   binding;   may   activate complements production.

CELLULAR IMMUNITY:

T lymphocytes mediate cellular immunity, against viruses, fungi, and intracellular bacteria. They are also immune- regulatory on other cells of the immune system. They arise from the bone marrow but mature in the thymus where they acquire specificity before they leave the thymus to populate other lymphoid organs.

T lymphocytes can be segregated into two subsets on basis of their functions
CD8 (cytotoxic) T lymphocytes. They destroy cancerous cells, viruses infected cells and allografts. Their actions are selectively specific.
CD4 + (Helper) T lymphocytes; They stimulate production of cytotoxic T cells which destroy antigen presenting cells. They also produce cytokines which support activation of CD8 + T lymphocytes.

The above functions of the immune system show that if we strengthen our immune system through our diets and lifestyles~ we can prevent and could cure our diseases including cancers.

The case of Mark Origer (2004) shows how the immune system works to defend the body. Conventional treatments had failed to cure his skin cancer (melanoma) which had metastasized (spread) to the liver. He was saved by genetic engineering of his immune system. His immune cells were taken from his body, which were given a gene that programmed them to attack melanoma cells. They survived and destroyed his tumour. Only Mark and one other man (out of 17 patients) responded in the trial. Mark's tumours are gone and he is cancer free. (Nig. Guardian 06/09/07.) Scientists taught the immune system to identify cancer cells, attack and destroy them. British scientists are working on an approach which involves taking T-cells, which fight infection and giving them ability to recognize a special tag on cancer cells called the WT1 protein and by so doing kill the cancer cells.

When genetic engineering is improved many deadly diseases could be cured by strengthening the immune system. This is how our diet, lifestyles, which strengthen our immune system could be the prevention and cure of our non-communicable diseases including cancers.

CHAPTER TWO

ACTIVITIES THAT AFFECT OUR STATE OF HEALTH, OXIDATION, FREE RADICALS, ANTI-OXIDANTS

Today, much scientific attention is being directed at the study of wear and tear of living organisms, breathing and eating. These nonstop activities place continuous stress on every cell of the body. The cell must fight back otherwise it suffers severe damage or be killed.

Every cell of the body is a biological machine that is gradually torn down by the work of staying alive. However, it is also an imperfect machine which does not have "100 percent efficiency."

Like the machine, the cell uses food nutrients and oxygen, at great price, to produce energy. This process of using oxygen is called OXIDATION. A neutral oxygen molecule consists of equal numbers of protons, in the nucleus, which are positively charged and electrons, which are negatively charged. The electrons are located in orbits around the nucleus, where the protons are located.

FORMATION OF FREE RADICALS

During oxidation, an oxygen molecule could lose one of its electrons, leaving it positively charged. This positively charged particle is known as OXYRADICAL or FREE RADICAL or REACTIVE OXYGEN SPECIES (ROS) or BIOLOGICAL BAD BOYS. These ROS are very unstable and highly reactive, in an attempt to return to their neutral state. These free radicals can react with minerals such as iron to form the highly dangerous HYDROXYL FREE RADICALS. They have the potential of causing damage to the cell membranes, its fats and its proteins. They cause cell death (apoptosis) with the disruption of RNA and DNA patterns. This disruption leads to Non Communicable Disease (NCD) e.g. cancers heart diseases, inflammations in joints, brain degradation, diabetes, auto-immune disorder and senility (aging). This process of damaging structures by free radicals is known as oxidative stress. Thus causing senility and many other age related diseases. Ageing is a consequence of continuous attack on our cells by free radicals. (GSH by Gutman, Jimmy). Those who live 100 years or more have high levels of glutathione, which counter the effects of free radicals.

The harmful effects of these ROS are countered by another substance in the body which supplies the ROS with an electron to neutralize the molecule. The supplier of this electron is the ANTIOXIDANT. The body's principal antioxidant is Glutathione assisted by others like Vitamin A, C, E and selenium. When the antioxidants are in short supply the free radicals wreak havoc on the cells. The antioxidant levels are improved by healthy live foods and food supplements.

FREE RADICALS IN THE BODY
They oxidize several blood constituents including harmful Low Density Lipoproteins (LDL) which are deposited on artery walls. These oxidative injuries arising from the effects of free radicals or reactive oxygen species (ROS) are the fundamental mechanisms underlying a number of degenerative disorders.

SOURCES OF FREE RADICALS / REACTIVE OXYGEN SPECIES (ROS)

Each time the immune system is threatened from the internal or the external environment, free radicals are released. They are produced by
our activities
and poor diet
 Frying produces lots of free radicals by producing undesirable alterations in the chemical compositions of oils and fats. Prolonged heating of unsaturated fats also produces toxic substances, polymerized products, peroxides and plenty of free radicals. These are the reasons why we must not fry foods because it can also make the food carcinogenic (Causing cancer). Foods heated above body temperature start-losing their nutritive and biological values. Frying (usually with oil raises the temperature of the food to about 130 ^{o}C). At such a temperature, Vitamins, co-enzymes, flavonoids are destroyed.
We can then imagine what happens to the food at this temperature. The following are the effects of frying foods.

·   The Food now has high fat content
·   Chemical decomposition of oil occurs; breaking long chain unsaturated fats into shorter chain fatty acids.
·   Acrolein is formed during frying. This irritates the gut mucosa-causing leaky gut. It could also be carcinogenic.
 Other sources of free radicals include
Improperly managed and excessive exercises.
Excessive stress
Air pollution
Cigarette smoking and smoke inhalation by non-smokers
Illnesses/infections
Medicines and ultra violet rays
Acidic and impure water

Microwave ovens
Burns
Overhead wirings and
Alcohols

ANTIOXIDANTS

Our cells are naturally equipped with antioxidants that neutralize free radicals by giving them the missing electrons. These oxidative damages caused by free radicals could be minimized by raising the level of natural antioxidants; glutathione and others, derived from our natural foods. A good store of these antioxidants, keep the free radicals in check.

SOURCES OF ANTIOXIDANTS

The body has its store. Anti-oxidants are also abundant in fruits and vegetables. Coloured fruits and vegetables; yellow, orange and green are the principal sources of antioxidants and micronutrients. Onions and garlic are very good sources of antioxidants. Damage caused by free radicals can therefore be overtaken by eating plenty of fruits and vegetables which have plenty of antioxidants.

Eating carrots, oranges, lettuce, grapes, tomatoes, cutting down on sugars and fats and avoiding other free radical sources mentioned above, exercising regularly, saves one from considerable damage by free radicals thus averting chronic diseases and cancers.

The most important external antioxidants include: Beta-carotenes, vitamins A, C and E. Others are selenium, chromium, zinc and calcium. These antioxidants act synergistically with glutathione, enhancing each other's effectiveness. Vitamins A, C and E pick up free radicals and hand them over to glutathione.

The positively charged (O+) oxygen radical is given an electron by glutathione to form O2. The glutathione now pairs with another radicalized glutathione to form a neutral nontoxic GSSG.

Selenium is an important part of the enzyme glutathione peroxidase. Because of this, it is said to be a glutathione booster and a good antioxidant. It picks up and supplies cysteine used in production of glutathione. Selenium has been linked with prevention and treatment of many chronic diseases, cancers and heart diseases. It fights these diseases by raising glutathione peroxidase levels in the cells. It is found in whole grain cereals, particularly wheat germ and bran, also, onions, garlic and mushrooms.

Other co-factors for glutathione production are vitamins C, B1, B2, B6, B12 and folic acid. Vitamin B6 contributes to over 60 enzyme systems. Folic acid takes part in a number of processes including DNA synthesis and neurotransmission. Zinc contributes to glutathione levels in the body.

Quercetin (useful antioxidant), abundant in red apples, red onions, berries, cabbages, broccoli and green and black tea, is believed to have multiple antioxidant and anti-inflammatory and cell energy activation properties that benefit health.

Many antioxidants in food are recognized by their distinctive colours like the deep red of cherries, tomatoes, apples, the orange colour of carrots, the yellow colour of corn and mangoes, the blue-purple of blue berries, black berries and grapes. Beta-carotenes abound in these fruits.

Many cancers and degenerative diseases are preventable and, possibly, remission is possible using plant derived substances

found in healthy diet. Young people produce enough antioxidants to mop up their free radicals. Older people do not produce enough antioxidants that can mop up the free radicals they produce. The free radicals are therefore available to ravage the unsaturated (F.A) acids on RBC membranes converting them to peroxides and aldehydes which are risk factors for cancers (Nigeria Guardian 11/08/10)
Phytochemicals are Plant chemicals which God has designed to serve the dual purpose of providing protection to both plants and man.

EXERCISE
Exercise is one of the essentials of healthy living. Others are water, air, salt and natural food.

Before now, medical experts have associated inactivity and obesity to four non communicable diseases. These are cancers, stroke, heart attack and complications of diabetes which reduce the life expectancy and life span of any individual. Today, physical activities appear to be associated with reduced, slower progression to the above age-related diseases as well as improved health in old age. This means that exercise has a clinically relevant impact on age-related diseases and boosts life expectancy. (Achieves of int. medicine 25/01/10)

Life expectancy is the number of years lived in good health. Exercise produces significant less erosion of telomeres on chromosomes, thus its anti-aging effects at the cellular levels especially in the cardiovascular system and the brain. Telomeres are strands of DNA at the tip of chromosomes known as biological caps associated with aging. Telomeres ensure that each DNA replication is completed (circulation of JAMA). They reduce in size as the cells divide causing DNA to become damaged and raising the odds of age-related diseases. Cells die after 60-100 divisions. Doctors have now found out that physical activity results in increased capacity which leads to many health benefits.

Recent studies show that exercise stimulates the production of a protein called Vascular Endothelial Growth Factor (VEGF) which encourages growth of new vessels (angiogenesis) in the muscles. (Cardelia J.A. L.S.U. HL.SC. Centre)

Effects of exercise in the body include:
- Reduces stress
- Improves muscle strength and muscle pumps, thus,
- Improves blood circulation.
- Improves cardiovascular risk factors in addition to fibrinolysis which improves endothelial function and decreases sympathetic tone.
- Opens up capillaries in muscles and by lowering resistance to the blood flow in arteries, lowers blood pressure, thus reducing cardiovascular risk.
- Improves body immune system by increasing circulation of natural killer (NK) cells that fight bacteria, viruses and cancer.
- Increases Natural Killer cell, (NK cell). These are a type of lymphocyte, able to kill viruses infected cells and cancerous cells and mediates in rejection of bone marrow grafts. By their actions above, form part of natural immunity.
- Improves filtration in kidneys resulting in the elimination of toxins and free radicals. This is why we are encouraged to drink a good quantity of water before exercising so as to increase urine output.

- Encourages the activities of fat burning enzymes for production of energy for muscular activities, thus reducing fat store with resultant weight loss. One hour walking causes activation of fat burning enzymes for 12 hours. Morning and evening walks activate the enzymes for 24 hours.
- Hydrates and oxygenates the organs very well which is a sure step to cancer, prevention and cure.
- Helps to preserve tryptophan and tyrosine which are precursors of neurotransmitters in the brain. They also play a role in the enzyme system that repairs incorrect DNA transcriptions. Tryptophan is used by the brain to manufacture serotonin, melatonin, tryptamine and indolamine which are antidepressants and regulate sugar levels and blood pressure.
- Builds up muscle mass by preventing muscles from being burnt as fuel.
- Enhances insulin sensitivity in the muscles, thus reducing hypoglycemic medications. Unexercised muscles are broken down-disuse atrophy. This causes loss of zinc and vitamin B which results in some neurological and autoimmune disorders.
- Strengthens bones, thus helps prevent osteoporosis.
- Decreases risk of orthopedic injuries.
- Clears cholesterol deposits in the arteries by decreasing total Low Density lipoprotein (LDL-Bad cholesterol) and increasing High Density Lipoprotein (HDL, good cholesterol).
- Improves mental alertness.
- Reduces the risk of breast and colon cancers.
- Elevates antioxidant enzymes and cofactors
- Antioxidant levels are inversely related to mortality (GSH-Gutman Jimmy).

- Single best therapy for peripheral Artery Disease (PAD) (Guardian 7/01/10)

World cancer research fund scientists suggest that 45 minutes a day of moderate exercise could prevent 5,500 cases of breast cancer.

It is advisable that our doctors advise us on our personal exercise tolerance levels. Ideally, we should exercise daily or at least 5 times a week, for 20-30 minutes as our heart performances allow. Our daily exercise should include stair climbing, brisk walking, gardening, swimming or cycling. Walking and cycling should be done in the open or in gardens where we breathe fresh oxygen. It is obvious today that the concentration of oxygen in the air is less due to environmental pollution as a result of industrialization, gas flaring in the Niger Delta, carbon monoxide from automobiles etc. Exercises in the gymnasia should be left for the athletes. Walking, uses almost all the 206 bones and 660 muscles of the body.

World Cancer Research Fund says; about one third of the most common cancers are preventable through a nutritious diet, maintaining a healthy weight and regular physical exercises. Healthy food and exercise could cut cancer rates by 90 percent. Simple changes in diet and exercise can prevent nearly 40 percent of breast and pancreatic cancers, 36 percent of lung cancers, over 60 percent of mouth cancers and 45 percent of bowel cancers. By adding vitamin D, which by itself has been demonstrated to prevent 77 percent of all cancers, cancer prevention rate approaching 90 percent can easily be achieved. The report did not mention elimination of dangerous cancer causing chemicals from diet such as sodium nitrite found in processed meats and artificial sweeteners.

Sixty scientific studies suggest that women who exercise regularly have 20-30 percent reduction in chance of getting breast cancer. Studies have also shown that while the metropolitan Chicago woman weighs 83.6 Kg, a Nigerian, rural farmer woman weighs 57.7kg. This is because the Nigeria women's diet consists of high fibre and carbohydrates, low in fat and animal protein. The Nigeria women spends most of her day in the farm. In contrast, the Chicago diet is 40-50 percent fat and high in processed foods with no farming activities. (Loyola Univ. Health System).

A study of 300 women on treatment for breast cancer showed that those with hormone responsive tumours who walked for 3-5 hours a week, at average pace, reduced their risk of dying from that disease by 50 percent compared to sedentary women. It has also been shown that regular exercise and drinking green tea may play an important role in prevention of depression among breast cancer survivors.

Hypertension and other chronic diseases that lead to kidney failure were on the increase in Nigeria because most of us now consume unhealthy "fast food," cigarettes and alcohols but do not exercise.

It should also be noted that exercise produces lots of free radicals due to increased muscle activities, but most of these are excreted through profuse sweating and increased kidney filtration rates.

It should be noted therefore that exercise is one of the pillars on which healthy life stands.

Regularly active adults are less likely to develop colon, liver; pancreatic and stomach cancers. The protective effects were more significant in men and women of normal weight.

Exercise has been shown to restore stem cell growth, and improve behavior in young mice that suffered brain damage induced by clinical radiation. It is therefore believed that children, who suffer similar brain damage by radiation, will benefit immensely from exercise.

Most active men are 15 percent less likely to develop cancer than least active men, while most active women have 16 percent lower cancer risk than their sedentary counterparts. These results are true when other factors age, weight, smoking habits, daily calorie intake are accounted for.

HIGH INTENSITY TRAINING (HIT) This is an alternative to the usual long exercise. It lasts few minutes but it's able to achieve much. It appeals to most busy people. This consists of running flat out for one minute then jogging for 2-3 minute before doing another one minutes sprint. This cycle is repeated 10 times.

FASTING AND PRAYER
Fasting is defined as the absence of caloric intake for 8 hrs. It could be partial or complete when even water is not taken for a period. Medically, this is limited to abstinence from foods and beverages in our daily menu and staying on water or homemade vegetable juices. Religiously, fasting is denying oneself some basic comfort, so that one can get that which he is asking from God. Fasting and prayers are aimed at seeking the face of God, to have divine audience with him. All major religions have prescribed periods of fasting and prayers. Lent for Christians and Jews, and Ramadan for Muslims. "What things so ever you

desire, when you pray, believe that you receive them and you shall have them" Mark 11:24. Faith and meditation will melt away the inner fears that have been eating into us.

Fasting and prayers have been scientifically proven to prevent illnesses, enhance psychological wellbeing and prolong life. However, fasting can be dangerous for people with diabetes, kidney diseases or heart diseases, pregnant women and children. Periodic fasting may well mean less disease and gain of years in the long run. The prayerful person reduces stress by his trust in God, believing that God gives him what he deserves with consequent reduction in the insatiable nature of man.

During fasting, toxins are rapidly released from their fat stores and with good water intake, are easily eliminated from the body. While toxins and free radicals excretions are going on, new ones from food are not produced. Energy needed by the body for digestion is re-directed to boosting immune system functions, cleansing body tissues, maintaining real weight, combating chronic ailments, improving mental health, as it reduces anxiety and decreases tension and educates taste buds. (Nig Guardian 01/04/10) Pressure on the immune system is subsequently reduced. If fasting is combined with enemas, it produces fantastic results even in cancer patients. The enema removes lots of toxins and free radicals.

Religious faithful, who fast, live healthier lives than care free individuals. They train themselves to eventually abstain from harmful foods, alcohols, smoking and correspondingly achieve weight control which enhances prolonged life; thus eliminating all risks associated with obesity. Those who attend Church, Mosque or Synagogues at least once a week are happier and have 40 percent lower blood pressure than those who do not (n

= 4,000 above 65 years in USA). They have greater life expectancy than non-believers living up to 14 years longer than nonbelievers. These better results may be due to these assumptions:

1.   If people believe that God protects and provides for them, they are likely to be optimistic and lead less stressful and therefore, healthier lives.
2.   If one waits on God by fasting and prayers, he lives a moderate lifestyle.
3.   We should avoid promiscuity. This results in reduced risk of contracting STDs, and social habits such as smoking of cigarettes/cannabis sativa and excessive drinking of alcohol.
Psychology plays the most fundamental part in divine healing.

When someone prays, he is invoking positive mental images which improve immune functions. Psychologists agree that prayer therapy is a most effective healing agent but prayer combined with fasting might be the single most important tool in the reconstruction of a person's personality.

Doctors should assist their patients with prayers always; healing will be faster and more efficacious. If the motto "God heals and we care" holds then all health providers must at certain times stop and pray for God's healing hands on their patients. Holistic medicine must involve God's grace and mercies. Evidences are now available to show that patients who pray do better than those who do not pray. The international Heart Collaboration in Utah shows her population has lowest rates of death from cardiovascular diseases in the USA. This may be connected to her highest population of church of Christ of Later Day Saints, who teach fasting from childhood. The findings showed Later Day

Saints adherents have lower heart diseases, 61% versus 77% in others. (Nig. Guardian 23/10/10).

MEDITATION AND FAITH IN GOD

These are necessary for reduction of stress. It is our insatiable quest today that saddles us with stress related diseases which shorten our life. During meditation, we conjure inner peace and tranquility to our inner self so we can commune with God. True physical healing begins with cleansing of our thoughts and feelings. We can then come to terms with God's goodness, come to trust and abandon ourselves to him and believe that he can cure us of our diseases and cancer. Remember, "I am the Lord the one who heals you" (Gen 15:26); "He forgives all my sin and heals me of my diseases" (Ps 103:2): That faith in God "heals" is a reality that must be taken seriously by both orthodox and complementary medicine practitioners. Faith and meditation will melt away life's inner fears and negative thoughts that have been eating into us. **"He will keep you safe from all hidden dangers and from all deadly diseases"** (Psalm 91:3)

REST

The body needs adequate rest to allow for its regeneration. During rest, there is reduction in production of free radicals and removal of already produced ones. Good night rest increases hormonal production. Late night meals reduce rejuvenation time and resting for the intestines and other body organs.

Vital to having a healthful lifestyle is getting the right quantity of sleep. During sleep, the body rebuilds itself and recuperates, getting ready for another day of activities. The following can help us have good rest:

1.   Vigorous exercise during the day in fresh air and sunlight.

2.   Adopt a night-time routine, e.g. a warm bath or doing some quiet reading.

3.   Avoid stimulating things such as television and stressful conversations.

4.   Do not over react or have heavy evening meals.

When digestion is not completed before sleep, the digestive process continues during sleep resulting in unpleasant dreams.

5.   Refrain from tobacco, nicotine, caffeine or alcohol.

6.   As much as possible, resolve unfinished businesses before bedtime.

7.   Have regular hours of sleep. Early to bed early to rise. The deepest sleep occurs between 9.00pm and 12.00 midnight.

8.   Have abundant supply of fresh air in your bedroom while asleep.

9.   Start your sleep by lying supine (face up) spreading your hands by your sides.

This fully relaxes all muscles making your rest worthwhile.

10 .God has asked us to rest on the Lord's Day. We should avoid secular duties so as to relax ourselves for the next week's activities.

LOVE

True love of God and our fellow men is a powerful healer. There is no feeling of resentment against another man and God. This gives inner peace. Love changes the chemical pathways in the brain positively and improves resistance to diseases. Health care providers must show empathy and sincerity to their patients as this is very effective if not more effective than the legion of prescriptions. A smile, when in difficulty, or to the sick can affect life positively for you or another person and can add to your life span or to that of your patients.

Love is a powerful healer, giving or receiving it. Diseases are aggravated when no one shows love to a patient. There is a popular saying "Love to a patient does not heal diseases but cools the heart". If they have someone, who shows love, they open up their complaints so lets off steam from their body. This definitely improves patient's symptoms. The bible tells us to love our neighbor as we love ourselves. Love across all religions, sex and nationality is what our creator wants from us. God said: if you do not love your neighbor whom you see, how can you love me whom you do not see. (Obesity, cancer depression by Batmanghelidj)

SMILE
Releases very friendly chemicals that positively boast the immune system.
Aborts stress and calms the nerves even if forced on an individual Communicates love to you and people around. A smile to the sick makes him return which lifts his spirit positively.
Gladdens the heart in he that smiles and those around him clinicians and other health care providers should always smile to their patients not minding their disposition at the time.

LAUGHTER
This has similar effects as love on the immune system. Periodic laughter is now being used as additional therapeutic measure in Europe. Barbara Rutting recommends that people laugh forcefully several times a day to boost their immune system.

SUNLIGHT

The energy of sunlight is good for healing. It helps to correct osteoporosis and rickets. Its implication in skin cancer is due to over-exposure. It converts cholesterol on the skin to vitamin D and encourages storage of Adenosine Triphosphate (ATP) energy in the bone. Vitamin D also encourages absorption of calcium from the intestine. Thus it is beneficial in treatment of high blood pressure and cancers.

Calcium has a balancing effect on the cell PH thus alleviating asthmatic complications.

GRATITUDE

Give up resentment and anger as these depresses the immune system. Fill your mind with good things. Multiply gratitude for any good done to you no matter how small.

MUSIC

Do not neglect the healing effect of music. Classical, harmonious and religious music translate into internal harmony of the body, exerting strong healing effects. Soft, happiness generating music should be used as a treatment protocol in disease treatment especially cancers. Let soft classical or religious music of patient's choice filter into the ears of the very ill and watch his reactions.

Masaru Emoto, an outstanding Japanese scientist has shown that water reacts to what it hears. When we remember that our body is about 75% water; the influence of harmonious sound can translate into inner harmony of our body. This exerts a strong healing influence on our body.

TEMPERANCE

Temperance is strict adherence to those things that promote health. This involves the elimination of such harmful things as alcohol, tobacco, drugs, caffeinated drinks, fatty foods and refined sugar. This definition is claimed by modernists as old fashioned. They regard temperance as controlling what you eat to moderation and not abstinence. Who measures the individual moderation limit? One hundred years ago, the average American consumed about 18kg of table sugar per year, today its 46kg. Refined sugar adds empty calories to our diet and destroys the body's ability to fight off bacteria. Regular 35c1 soda (soft drink) contains 8-10 teaspoons of sugar which decreases the ability of white blood cells to fight bacteria by 50%. Tragically American youths today drink more soft drinks than pure water.

NATURAL FRESH AIR
This has become a rare commodity today especially in the urban cities of our developing countries. Here, there are no restrictions to siting of industries within residential areas, disposal of industrial and household wastes, and gas flaring as in oil producing communities. The rejected automobiles of the developed countries have taken over our roads injecting into the air unquantifiable quantities of carbon monoxide and nitric oxide. At night when some industrial machines are silent and most automobiles are packed, evil doers take over, making it impossible for evening and night road walks in gardens. Personal houses in developed and developing "countries, used to have beautiful gardens decorated with different flowers that produce oxygen. These have given way to houses with high rise block fences where we can hardly see the ground floor of the buildings behind, especially in developing countries because of insecurity.

We need fresh air that contains ions which promote the wellbeing of our bodies.

Let us stay outside in the evenings and night to receive fresh air. Keep windows open to allow fresh air with its high quality oxygen needed by red blood cells especially during rest.

Today, more and more people are concerned with the quality of air they breathe. The pollution in the air decreases the amount of oxygen that actually gets to the lungs and blood. A prevalent ingredient in polluted air-carbon monoxide, binds with oxygen in the blood, making it ineffective. Many are dying each year from air pollution.

MICROWAVES

Microwaves are electromagnetic waves that are shorter than radio waves but longer than light waves. There are generated by the oscillations of electrons in electronic devices. There are two types of micro waves.

(a)   Ionizing radiation. These waves agitate and split the atom

(b)   Non ionizing radiation can't split the atom but agitates the molecules. Scientifically these molecular agitations cannot last for two long without harmful effects. General Service of Mobile Communication (GSM) which emits microwaves is only 25 years in existence. This is why Scientist caution on it uses. The radio frequency waves emitted from mobile phones have been shown to alter brain wave activity (JAMA Feb 2011). This study showed increased glucose metabolism (a sign of brain activity) in people exposed to cell phones in areas closest to the antenna. This finding lends credence to a previous study which suggested long term use of such devices may be implicated in brain cancer.

A Finish study (Int. Journal of cancer 2007) found a link between cell phone use and cancer. Depending on rate and duration of use, cell phone radiation was responsible for up to 27% incidence in gliomas - a type of brain tumour.

Nigeria Public Health scientists say the health hazards of modern electronic gadgets now endanger us 100 million times more than the case with our grandparents. (Nig. Guardians 10/03/11). They say closest culprit is the cell phones. Others include food processors, laptops, desktop computers, refrigerators microwave ovens, telecom masks, power lines, transformers, television sets, vacuum cleaners, hair dryers etc. These scientists say hazards due to these appliances "may threaten our very own existence on earth."

A recent World Health Organization (WHO) International Agency on cancer study (N: 10'751) in May 2010 indicates the dangerous connection of cancer cell development and frequencies and radiation emitted from cell phones. Children are one of the most vulnerable group to electro-pollution. Recent studies show 31% cancer increase in this age group (Nig. Guardian 10/03/11). This is why scientists caution on it uses. Microwave ovens cook food using electromagnetic waves instead of heat. Microwaves have carcinogenic effects on humans. The high speed oscillations (up to 5 billion times per sec) of microwaves in microwave pots/ovens cause considerable changes in the natural alignment of food particles. The different food substances, proteins, vitamins, carbohydrates, minerals etc., separate and are grouped in linear forms resulting in considerable alterations in the food molecules. Microwaves can have similar effects as in microwave ovens/pots on any tissue it is in contact with. Therefore long term exposure to microwaves such as use of cell phones, living below or near high tension electric lines, radio and phone towers should be avoided at all costs.

Do not carry your cell phones on your breast pockets and other sensitive areas of the body such as trouser/skirt pockets to avoid irradiating the testicles/ovaries.

FORGIVENESS

The brain chemistry is directly affected by forgiveness which has strong therapeutic effect on the brain and the body in general. Revenge converts constructive powers of the brain into negative energy of destruction.

When one thinks of revenge, the insult or injury which caused it is re-enacted in the body. This has a negative effect on the body because the brain chemistry will be engaged in these negative thoughts again and again. Remember that the physics theory of equal and opposite forces does not apply here. Consequently, you could put yourself into greater physical harm as you go to revenge. The Christian faith reminds us that "tit for tat" no longer applies. We should pray for our enemies and not "return to sender" the harm done to us.

Forgive the truck pusher who abuses you while on your steering, he may be reacting to the frustration not caused by you but by the "harsh" economic circumstances he finds himself at that time.

CHAPTER THREE

OUR DIET

This is the sum total of food consumed by a person.
Natural diet, oxygen and water formed the tripod on which life stands. This is why we should turn to natural foods as was consumed by our ancestors. "God has given you every seed bearing plant on the face of the earth and every tree that has fruit with seed in it. They will be yours for food" (Gen 1:29). Daniel ate fruits and vegetables without meat and was very healthy. In developing countries, non- communicable diseases are on the increase. In these countries eating processed food is considered as "one has arrived". Unfortunately, lack of education and poverty make it impossible for people of the poorer countries to take the measures that reduce the non-communicable diseases as in the developed countries.

The living body has the capacity to survive and reverse diseases including cancers if it depends on the tripod above. Our health status depends on what we give it. Given the right ingredients, it soars on, but given the wrong nutrients, it wobbles and fumbles along with non-communicable diseases including cancers till the exit date. In most cases, if the required body ingredients in food are given to it by change of our lifestyles and diet, health is restored and the body normalizes and remissions of diseases take place. If you return to your former lifestyle, you reap the same harvest as before; non-communicable, chronic diseases and cancers. Prof. Augustine Ohovoriole, the president of the Nigerian Society of Endocrinology and metabolism recently said there is already an epidemic of non-communicable diseases in Nigeria due to Western diet or refined foods and inactivity.

Natural food is designed by our creator in forms that have enough of our body needs because they are natural stores of antioxidants which fight non-communicable diseases and cancers. If we wish to recover, from any disease, cancer in particular to remain healthy, eat fresh foods or half boiled if possible.

Kansas State University researchers have developed a branch of studies known as NUTRIGENOMICS, which combines molecular biology, genetics and nutrition to regulate gene expressions through food nutrients. This gives new hope to present and future cancer patients whose treatments will be based on what they eat as proclaimed in this small book. World Cancer Research Fund estimates that diet is responsible for about 35-60% of all forms of cancers.

Studies have shown that Mediterranean diet might be the secret to living longer and healthier lives. The diet consists of grapes, red wine, olive oil, peanuts, plant-based foods and restricted calories. When exercise is added to this food, longevity further improves.

The active ingredient in red wine and grape is RESVERATROL which is a flavonoid. Moderate wine drinkers are known to have less risk for dementia, stroke and other cardiovascular diseases. Resveratrol has high antioxidant effects.

It is agreed by all health care providers that foods such as sea foods, fruits, vegetables, green tea, nuts, unpolished grains, legumes, onions, ginger, garlic, green pepper, olive oil, moderate alcohol, foods high in vitamins A, C and E and beta-carotene contribute a lot to healthy lives.

Swapping fried and salty foods for fruits and vegetables could cut the global incidence of heart attack by 33 percent. The typical western diet, high in fat, salt and meat, accounts for about 30 percent of heart attack risks in any population.

The time has come when our foods should be the simplest type and mildly cooked. Self-denial must be practiced in regard to those foods that are not good for the body, so that we do not eat that which satisfies the appetite but injures the digestive system and the body in general. It is difficult and almost impossible for an intemperate person in diet to exercise patience and self-control. Gluttons beware.

Herein are suggestions on healthy diet.
1.   Boil or steam, rather than fry foods.
2.   Eat raw foods at every meal. Avoid salad dressings that are high in fat.
3.   Eat fresh or dried fruits for dessert instead of junk foods.
4.   Avoid between meals or snacks. Snacking shuts down on going digestion to start another.
5.   Eat slowly to allow digestion start in the mouth and prevent overeating because taste buds are   not satisfied.
6.   Set a daily time table; to eat, exercise, rest and try to keep to it.

MALNUTRITION
This is the condition caused by an improper balance between what an individual eats and what he requires to maintain good health. This results from taking too little, excess or incorrect balance of basic foodstuffs or a deficiency of one of the many

minerals and vitamins which the body requires to be in good health.

1)   Obesity can be said to be one of the signs of malnutrition. Others are: Marasmus and kwashiorkor. In Obesity, excess fat is accumulated mostly in the subcutaneous tissues where it might have negative effects on health. Obesity is said to occur when body mass index (BMI) is 30 or above.

$$BMI = \frac{\text{Weight in Kilogram}}{(\text{Height in metres})^2}$$

BMI: above 30 is obesity; 25-29 is overweight; 18-24 is normal; less than 18 is underweight.

Obesity reduces life expectancy by7.1years in men and 5.8 in women among non-smokers and 13.7 years and 13.3 years respectively among smokers.

While coronary disease is major cause of death among the obsessed, cancer rates are also increasing in the overweight especially colorectal cancer in males and cancer of gallbladder, biliary tract, breast endometrium and cervix in females. (Davidson's principles & practice of medicine, 20th edition Pg.111)

2)   Marasmus: This is a mixed deficiency of both proteins and calories resulting in severe wasting of infants   whose
weight may fall 60% below that accepted for their age. The child lacks skin fat. It is community seen in war torn developing countries and in famine.

3)   Kwashiorkor: This is a form of malnutrition mostly due to a diet deficient in proteins. It is also seen in infants and children in very poor communities, war torn developing countries and during famine. Here, the child has edema, with loss of appetite,

diarrhea and very pale with puffy face, pot belly and chances in hair colour.

Unlike marasmus and kwashiorkor, obesity is due to consumption of more food than is required for a healthy living. While genetic elements may be involved, control of one's diet to a large extent controls his weight.

Obesity is already an epidemic in the USA where nearly 30 percent of the adult population are obsessed and 20 percent in the UK. The children are not left out even in the developing countries. This is fueled by "Junk foods" from fast food shops located on every corner of the streets. Their tastes, smells and low prices make them most handy for all classes of people. Children's parties are not celebrated without cakes, ice creams, candies and soda drinks, while adult tea breaks are filled with fast foods. These are high calorie foods which over load the body than it needs. The excess is stored in fatty tissues, thus resulting in obesity.

It is now well established that the risks of developing hypertension, heart diseases, arthritis, type 2 diabetes, stroke, cancers and other chronic debilitating diseases are very high in obese people.

It is unfortunate that through advertisements, feeding habits of children and adults alike are now being manipulated by beverage industries thereby loading us with excess calories. Complications of obesity include --- type 2 diabetes, hypertension, stroke, coronary heart diseases, diabetic complications, hormone dependent cancers etc. In all, obesity reduces life expectancy by 7.1 years in men and 5.8 years in women nonsmokers and by 13.7 years in men and 13.3 years in women respectively among smokers.

THE DIGESTIVE SYSTEM:

The digestive system is greatly injured by a large quantity of cold food and cold drinks because the body uses part of her energy to bring them to body temperature. Foods should therefore not be taken too hot or too cold. Water drank with meals diminishes production of saliva thus impairing digestion. Eat slowly so that saliva can mix well with food. This aids digestion. Do not take a great variety of food at the same time. Food should be cooked simply with such nicety which will invite the appetite.

The digestive system needs rest after each meal; a minimum of 5-6 hours should lapse between the meals. This is why two meals a day are better than three. Water, home-made fruit juices and vegetables could be taken between the meals at regular intervals (so called snacks or tea breaks).

Intestine: Inadequate emptying of the colon (large intestine) plays a, significant role in cancer formation (carcinogenesis). Food residues do not leave the colon early which results in reabsorption of toxic wastes. This stagnation is because we do not drink enough water. Good intake of water helps empty the bowel easily. Dr. Don Colbert said "we have created a lifestyle that is so toxic that we too have become toxic and is killing us (Nig. Guardian 28/8/08)

Cancer risks are reduced if we empty our bowels more than once daily.

Don't eat between meals so as to allow reasonable period for the intestines to rest.

Late night meals should be avoided.
Banana is an alternative to ice cream.

The large intestine harbors many useful bacteria called probiotics. A balance between them and harmful bacteria affect our longevity. The harmful bacteria cause "leaky" gut which results in reabsorption of toxins and carcinogens from the gut. The harmful bacteria also impair the immune system.

Probiotics:
- Produce antibodies against harmful bacteria.
- Synthesize Vitamin B complex and Vitamin K.
- Reduce blood bad cholesterols (LDL) and triglycerides.
- Maintain the integrity of the gut.
- Detoxify carcinogens in the gut and help maintain estrogen hormone balance.

For the afore mentioned reasons, special attention should be paid to our intestines especially the colon and rectum through the use of enemas and fasting.

ENEMAS
This is the use of fluids to cleanse the rectum (lowest part of the intestine).

Fluid is put in an enema can and connected to a tube (nozzle) which is inserted into the anus with the patient lying head down, with the elbows and knees on the bed. The anus is lubricated with K.Y jelly or aloe- Vera jelly.

Enema could be

(A) Cleansing enema that flushes the colon and the rectum thus removing feces and toxins.

(B) Retention enema which is primarily to help the liver and other organs eliminate their toxic. Either of them used during fasting makes detoxification more infective. In cleansing enemas, 3 lemon fruit juice and 2 litre of water are mixed.

The patient then lies on his back, then rolls over and lies on his left side. The fluid is allowed to stay in rectum for a few minutes. Deep breathing can help relieve any pains while the fluid is in the rectum.

Plain water can also cleanse the colon and rectum but not as good as lemon juice. (Dr Aiyesimoju, A. Nig. Guardian 28/08/08)

FRUITS

Fruits, nuts and berries have many antioxidants. They make the body alkaline which is preferred to acidity. The antioxidants in fresh fruits prevent the damage caused by free radicals. Don't let a day pass by without fruits or their home made juices.

In grains, fruits, vegetables and nuts are found all food elements we need. They constitute the food chosen for us by God (Gen 2:29). When cooked in a simple and natural manner are most nourishing foods for our bodies. Studies show that vegetarians are less likely to fall prey to cancer by at least one third.

Walnut: Walnuts are important sources of mono-unsaturated fats, polyunsaturated fats and antioxidants. They also contain the amino acid arginine which is a raw material for the production of nitrous oxide which relaxes arteries and keeps platelets from sticking on endothelial linings. They are rich in omega 3 (alpha linoleic acid) and omega 6 (linoleic acid). These are the essential fatty acids. These amino acids cannot be synthesized by the body and must be supplied by our diet because they are required by the body. Walnuts are also good sources of proteins and vitamins B1, B6, and folate. Omega 3 can reduce bad cholesterol (LDL), improve atherosclerosis and stabilize heart rhythm during heart attacks. Walnuts provide more omega 3 than any other food.

Essential fatty acids (EFA) are also available in oily fish (sardine, salmon and mackerel) and shellfish, soya oils, pumpkin seeds and leafy vegetables. The essential fatty acids are needed for adequate nervous system development. Other components of nuts that reduce heart diseases and cancer are fibre, phytosterols and flavonoids.

Nuts contain sterols which interfere with cholesterol absorption. Its essential fatty acids, antioxidants and phytosterol content reduce the risk of, and even cure, breast cancer. The African walnut also has antimicrobial effects against candida, staphylococcus, aspergillus and pseudomonas.

Soybean: Soybean is one of the legumes. It contains isoflavones which act similarly to the estrogen hormones and may have anti-cancer qualities in hormone-related cancer of the breast and prostate. Cells in lungs also have properties which suggest they also respond to isoflavonoids. It also contains protease inhibitors that may inhibit proliferation of cancer cells.

Soybean, like all legumes, contains genistein which is a cancer preventive nutrient and also an anti-clotting agent and thus prevents heart attacks and stroke. Other good sources of genistein include English pea and tofil. Women who eat more soy based foods have low risk of uterine and ovarian cancers. These cancers are affected by estrogen hormone which is mimicked by compounds in soy. The risk may be 40% lower among those who eat more soy. Soy is proven to be a heart protector. (Nig. Guardian 10/09/09).

"Soybeans contain phytochemicals which play a role in lowering cholesterol and countering heart diseases. They contain multiple cancer-fighting compounds. Genistein, found in soy, has ability to block development of cancer at different stages. There is hardly a dimension of disease process in which it does not hold potential to play a preventive role. That is true for diabetes, gall bladder and kidney stones, PMS (Post-Menopausal Syndrome) and menopausal symptoms, high blood pressure, heart diseases and cancers. The type of fibre and proteins which soybeans contain, added to their rich array of plant chemicals, make the soybean a unique and potent contributor to a host of health benefits" (Environmental Nutrition May, 1994. Vol. 17, No5). It contains isoflavones which act similarly to estrogen hormones and may have anti-cancer qualities in hormones related cancers breast and prostate (Guardian 11/02/10).

PINEAPPLES: Pineapples contain the enzyme bromelain, a sulfur rich protolithic enzyme known for its anti-tumor-properties and may also have anti-metastatic effects. It also has anti-clotting properties which help prevent ischemic strokes and heart attack. Pineapple has been shown to reduce swelling; help fight against sore throat, treat arthritis and gout and speeds the digestion of proteins. New research shows that pineapple is very effective at cancer prevention and treatment (Cancer letter 30/03/10)

The Indian Institutes of Toxicology researches have shown the anti-inflammatory anti - invasive and anti- metastatic properties of bromelain found in pineapples.

Therapeutic doses of dietary supplements of bromelain put a rapid halt to inflammation and reduce excessive coagulation of blood.

Citrus: These include oranges, grapes, tangerines and lime. Members of the citrus family are rich in flavonoids such as beta carotene, lutein and lycopene. These constituents are antioxidants and anti-cancer agents. More than 600 carotenoids occur naturally but carotenes are the most widely known. Carotenes offer protection against lung, colorectal, breast, uterine and prostate cancers. Other foods rich in flavonoids include: apricots, carrots, squash and tomatoes in addition to other green foods.

Citrus also contain limonoids which also help fight cancers of the mouth, skin, lung, breast, stomach and colon. They also reduce bad cholesterol, (low density lipoprotein LDL). Flavonoids, in citrus, show great promise for prostate and lung cancers, and melanomas. Citrus fruits are natural sources of vitamin C, potassium and folate. Potassium works to maintain fluid balance. It is depleted by coffee and, tea. Potassium plays a key role in lowering blood pressure, subsequently heart attacks and stroke. Citrus fruits are good sources of fibre including soluble fibres. Citrus fruits are cholesterol free. People trying to lose weight should take plenty of citrus fruits and vegetables which have high fibre and water content.

Flavonoids and limonoids in citrus fruits and their peels are known to lower blood cholesterol (LDL) more than most prescription drugs without risk of side effects. (Nig. Guardian 14/04/05).

Carrot: Carrots are rich in beta carotenes and other carotenoids. People can reduce their risk of stroke by as much as 54 percent if they eat lots of fruits and vegetables that are rich in carotenes, vitamin C and E (Nig. Guardian 11/08/05).

A Harvard university study (n=87,245) showed that those who ate carrot (and to a lesser extent spinach) 5 times a week reduced their risk of stroke by 68 percent than those who ate 2 times a week.

Tomatoes: Tomato was first cultivated in Peru then Mexico. Today, they are everywhere.

Eating tomatoes daily reduces cancer by 50% and prevents heart attack. 10 servings of tomatoes per week reduced chances of prostate cancer by 33% (N = 50,000). The following ingredients in tomatoes make them indispensable in our diets.
- Lycopene: This is one of nature's most powerful antioxidants. It fights different diseases mostly cancers-prostate, pancreas, bowel and breast.
- Fibre: The fibre prevents diabetes, asthma, colon cancer and lowers cholesterol level in the blood.
- Vitamins A and C are antioxidants which fight free radicals, aging and soothe the skin and hairs and boost the immune system.
- Potassium, Vitamin B6, folate and niacin lower cholesterol, blood pressure and heart diseases.
- Vitamin K in tomatoes helps to build bones.
- Chromium and biotin help the body to process sugar and fats thus improving diabetes and nerve functions.

·   Riboflavin helps in energy metabolism and fights against headache and migraine.

Aim at eating tomatoes every day for the above benefits.

Tomatoes contain two phytochemicals- procounaric and clorogenic acids which are thought to combat cancer by disrupting the making of nitrosamines which work to turn normal cells cancerous. These two chemicals are also found in green pepper, pineapples, strawberries and carrot.

Black pepper: Curcumin derived from black pepper has been found to decrease the number of cancer stem cells and has no effect on normal differentiated cells. Cancer stem cells are the small number of cells within the tumour.

Therefore eliminating the stem cells is the key to controlling and treatment of cancer. People whose diets are rich in curcumin-tumeric have lower rates of breast, lung and colon cancers.

Bitter Kola (Garcinia Kola): Nigerian researchers have shown that bitter kola is showing great promise in the management of respiratory diseases including asthma. They have shown that the major phytochemical contents are xanthine and flavonoids. These compounds inhibit calcium influx and histidine release which are stimulated by IgE dependent ligands respectively. Nigerian researchers have validated the efficacy of bitter kola 0.5% in eye drops in preventing blindness in patients with open glaucoma. It is as effective as timolol. (Nig. Guardian 14/10/10.)

Other diseases where Garcinia Kola has shown great promise include gastritis, jaundice, and also as a purgative and for relieve of cough. Flavonoids protect against allergies, inflammation, free radicals and platelets aggregations.

Almost every fruit/vegetable from berries to yams, citrus and cucumbers contain flavonoids, another antioxidant and anti-carcinogen agents.

GRAPE FRUITS EXTRACT: Lagos University researchers have shown the uses of grape fruits extracts (Quarterly J. Of Hosp. Med, Adeneye, A. A. 2010)

(1) It contains a flavonoid called naringenin also found in all citrus, especially grape fruits which give its characteristic bitter taste.

(2) Grape fruits seed extract contains high levels of Vitamin C, E and polyphenolic flavonoids glycosides - hesperidin, neohesperidin and naringenin. These compounds are most powerful antioxidants.

3)   The seed extract showed significant dose related lowering effects on
a)   Fasting Blood sugar
b)   Cardiovascular disease risks
c)   Lipid parameters except HDL which was significantly elevated
d)   Significant weight loss.

These results lend support to potentials in the management of type 2 diabetes.

4)   Nigerians have also shown effectiveness of grape fruit seeds in treating urinary tract infections (UTI) (J. Of C.A.M. Oyelami, O. A. et al)

5)   Ontario Canada researchers have also shown that naringenin, found in concentrations above normal levels in grape fruits seed

a.   Make liver burn fats instead of storing them.

b)   Corrected elevations in triglycerides and cholesterol c) Prevented insulin resistance.

d)   Improves obesity irrespective of food consumed

Cancer protective fruits and vegetables

FRUITS	VEGETABLES
Blueberries	Spinach, Kale
Strawberries	Lettuce, Collard greens
Plum	Brussels, sprouts, cabbage
Oranges	Beans, peas, lentils
Grapes	Carrots, beet, potatoes
Apricots	Mustard
Orange juice	Garlic, Onions
Grape fruits	Tomatoes
Kiwifruits	Yams, Sweet potatoes
Raspberries	Mixed vegetables
Blackberries	Watermelon
Bananas	Bell peppers

(M.K Gupta.   Foods killing you)

FIBRES

Fibres are parts of our plant foods that are resistant to digestion in the human digestive system. They are also called roughages and found on the skin and parts of vegetables and fruits. Soluble fibres are found in fruits, legumes, nuts and some vegetables and oat bran. The insoluble fibres are found in whole grains, fruits, vegetables, and nuts. Whole grains contain essential fatty acids

(EFA) which serve as precursors to prostaglandins, an important component of cell membranes.

The types of fibre that exert cancer protective effects are those in which pentose sugars are abundant. These polymers are abundant in unrefined cereals and in most vegetables except potatoes. They help to form bulky stool because of their water holding capacity and by increasing the number of fecal bacteria. This effect may be by increasing fecal bulk and hence diluting any carcinogen present or by reducing length of stay in contact with the mucosa. Fibres reduce cancer risk by binding carcinogens in the intestines thus, providing a good environment for beneficial bacteria (Probiotics) to flourish.

Whole grains like corn, whole wheat, oats and brown rice exhibit a level of anticancer activity that is equal to, and even greater than, levels found in vegetables and fruits. Whole grains contain many potent antioxidants. They contain vitamins, minerals and fibres which are removed when polished. Refined cereals cause B1 (thiamine) depletion which results in irritability, digestive disorders, heart and muscle diseases. Populations who consume high fibre diets have lower risk of colon cancer.

It is found that women who consumed the most fibre from cereals, vegetables, and fruits had a 29-46% reduction in cancer risk compared to those who ate least amount of fibre. Cancer Research centre Hawaii says, the risk of endometrial cancer could be reduced by consuming plant-based foods, low in fat, high in fibre and rich in whole grains, vegetables, fruits and legumes especially soybeans.

Legumes, tofu and other soy products are rich in phytoestrogens which control levels of estrogen in the blood. These findings suggest that prevention of endometrial cancer will involve:

1)   Weight control through reduction of energy intake, especially from fat and protein.
2)   Increase of soy and fibre mostly from vegetables and fruits (American journal of epidemiology, 1997: 146(4) 294-306)

food sources of cancer fighting phytochemicals

PHYTOCHEMICAL	FOOD
Sianigrin	Brussels, sprouts
Sulphoraphone	Broccoli
Dithiolthiones	Broccoli
Resveratrol	Red grapes
PEITC	Watercress
Limonene	Citrus fruits
Allyl sulphides	Garlic, Onions
Isoflavonnes, saponins	Soybeans, legumes
Protease inhibitors	Soybeans, legumes
Ellagic acid	Grapes
Caffeic acid	Fruits

Common Sources of Fibre

Foods	Fibre(gm)%	Food	Fibre(gm)%
Whole wheat bread	2.1	Cauliflower	4.6
Whole wheat	4.3	Broccoli	5.2
Pita bread	6.3	Peas	6.7
Popcorn	5.2	Brussels sprout	7.0
Oatmeal	4.1	Sweet potatoes	7.7

Spaghetti	4.5	Lentils	10.3
Shredded wheat biscuit	2.2	Pinto beans	12.0
Apple with skin	2.8	Navy beans	15.4
Oranges	3.1	Egg	0
Raw blackberries	7.2	Meat	0
Pears (canned)	7.7	Milk	0
Raspberries	1.1	Cheese	0

(Vance Ferrell, International meat crisis)

Foods less in fibre include: cake, potato chips, white bread, noodles, meat, fish, fruit juice, ice cream and milk to name a few.

Other sources of fibre include: maize, brown rice, millet, soybean, beans, carrot, cucumber, cabbage, lettuce, spinach, potato with skin, guava, mango, citrus fruits, apple and banana.

Fibre foods help control diabetes by lowering the rate of glucose absorption from the gut thus reducing blood glucose levels.

Fibre helps in weight reduction and control. It contributes few calories, thus one is full when one has actually taken little calories. It delays absorption of carbohydrates and fats. High fibre diets are low fat diets and vice versa.

GREEN VEGETABLES AND THEIR ROLES IN FIGHTING CHRONIC DISEASES AND CANCER

Green vegetables contain lots of chlorophyll. Chlorophyll contains as much magnesium as haemoglobin contains iron. Chlorophyll has the ability to make the body alkaline which is healthier to the body than being acidic, because cancers prefer acidity. Green vegetables contain many vital elements of life such as Vitamins, minerals, proteins, essential un-saturated fats, antioxidants and phytochemicals. They are indispensable for the living body. They also contain beta-carotenes and DHA (docosa-hexa-enoic acid), fatty acids needed by the brain.

The protective powers of food and exercise are daily unfolding, thus enabling people to preserve their health through dietary daily choices. The essential step is to modify diets and lifestyles. We are exposed daily to oxidizing compounds and carcinogens but compounds-antioxidants, phytochemicals, found in vegetables and fruits help to limit free radical productions and DNA damage, thus lowering the incidence of various cancers. Because these plant pigments are anti-inflammatory and antioxidant, they reverse cell damage. People who therefore eat lots of them have reduced cancer risk. These plant pigments include: chlorophyll, carotenoids and bioflavonoids. Chlorophyll is a detoxifier and possibly an anticancer agent.

As has been noted earlier, more than 600 carotenoids occur naturally but carotenes are the most widely known. Carotenes offer protection against lung, colorectal, breast, uterine and prostate cancers. Foods rich in flavonoids include: apricots, carrots, citrus fruits, tomatoes, in addition to many green foods. Catechins are active against pathogens and are thus protective against cancers. Sulphur-containing foods include broccoli, sprouts, cabbage, cauliflower, mustard and turnips. Radishes contain many sulfur containing compounds as well as in-doles, subclass of phytonutrients that bind chemical carcinogens. They activate detoxification enzymes especially in the Gastro-intestinal tract. In-doles and related compounds promote metabolism of carcinogens and oestrogen balance which could reduce risk of estrogen related cancers, example breast cancers.

Sulfur compounds - disulfides and trisulfides are active ingredients in garlic oil and S-cysteine in crushed garlic. They inhibit human metabolism and enhance the immune system. They also have antifungal and antibacterial effects. These effects may be through the glutathione system.

Garlic and onions help prevent men from developing prostate cancers.

THE LILY FAMILY: Garlic and onion contain good quantities of sulfur compounds. They enhance glutathione S-transferase enzymes which the liver uses in detoxification of carcinogens. They contain allylic sulphide, which works on enzymes to detoxify carcinogens.

Allium (the lilies) also increases immune enhancing actions that include production of lymphocytes, cytokinesis release, phagocytosis and natural cell activities.

Nitrosamine compounds, formed in the small intestine as a result of breakdown of nitrates and nitrites, from meats, are acted on by garlic, reducing the risk of their inducing cancer formations. These two compounds are used as additives in processing of ham, sausages and other meat products.

Many natural spices have anti-inflammatory, anti-cancer properties. Extracts of bitter leaf inhibit breast cancer and lower blood glucose. A phytochemotherapy for cancer made from bitter leaf collected from Benin City has received USA patent 6849604. Another bitter leaf-based herbal anti diabetic medication has also received USA Patent 6531461.

Best foods to block, intercept and stifle cancer include: Garlic, cabbage, soybeans, onions, carrots, tomatoes, all green and yellow vegetables, fruits, especially citrus (Oranges, grapes, Tangerines, lemons), fatty fish and green tea.

Calorie-restricted diet and increased physical activity fight obesity, cancer and enhances life span.

Restricting the consumption of glucose reduce lung cancer cells. (Nig. Guardian 20/11/08)

Olive oil is effective against HER-2 positive breast cancer for which orthodox medicine offers little by way of tolerable treatment. (Nig. Guardian 04/02/10)

Phytochemicals: RESVERATROL in red wine and catechin in green, white and red teas also reduce our risk to inflammatory diseases, cancers and diabetes. The phytochemicals interfere with the transmission of messages across cells involved in inflammation and cancers.

Green Tea: Green tea protects the body against oxidation. It has substances that degrade carcinogens. It helps keep harmful LDL (Low density lipoproteins), bad cholesterol, down, HDL (High density lipoproteins) good cholesterol high in people with elevated cholesterol. Thus it helps to keep blood pressure low. The catechins found in green tea, prevent the development of prostate cancer in men with High Grade Prostate Intraepithelial Neoplasm (PIN). Green tea also helps sharpen vision in age related macular degeneration (AM D).

Aloe Vera: Drinking aloe Vera juice:
1.   Boosts immunity system against cancer and HIV/AIDS.

2.   Compounds in aloe- Vera have anti-viral effects.

3.   Kills cancer cells.

4.   Reduce the growth rate of tumour and helps with allergies.

5.   It also promotes growth of non-cancerous cells thus promoting cancer fighting properties.

6.   It is one of the most potent sources of antioxidants: vitamins, E, C and B12.

7.   Its antioxidants counter ageing processes.

8.   Aids digestion.

9.   Enhances clear skin.

10.   Reduces cholesterol levels thus reducing hypertension and cardiovascular diseases.

Excessive heating and industrial filtration destroys some of its essential enzymes and poly-saccharides. Therefore used as near nature as possible.

Nigerian researchers led by Prof. Olukemi Odukoya have confirmed the potential of 21 green leafy vegetables (GLV) in the cooked form as natural sources of antioxidants. These leafy vegetables include commonly eaten vegetables in all parts of Nigeria (see table below). They are abundant during the rains and are here for the purpose of curing us of many communicable diseases and cancers. No wonder Nigerian researchers on our natural foods and herbs say "for every disease and cancer that afflict us, there is a green leaf in our garden that can cure it" (Rev. Fr. Dodo. Nig. Guardian 04/02/10).

High consumption of these our natural, native vegetables containing phenolic antioxidants may slow down the process of degenerative diseases. Studies have repeatedly shown that low vegetable meals correlate with increasing colon and stomach cancers. These vegetables provide high amounts of carotene, ascorbic acid and micronutrients which play great roles in metabolism. These antioxidants create a balance between production and removal of potentially damaging reactive oxygen species (ROS) or Free radicals or oxy-radicals. Destroying free radicals help fight cancers, heart diseases, stroke and other immune compromising diseases.

The cooked forms of these 21 leafy vegetables offer cheap but reliable sources of antioxidants, micronutrients and other phytochemicals essential for good health. These are more bio-available from cooked vegetables probably because cooking breaks down the tough cell walls releasing these nutrients for easier absorption.

Another isothiocynates chemicals found in cabbage and turnips called PEITC, for short, inhibit lung cancer by breaking carcinogens into fragments before they bind to cell's DNA. A phytochemical in strawberries, grapes and raspberries called ellagic acid also neutralizes carcinogens before they can invade DNA.

BROCCOLI

Broccoli and its relatives are nutritional power houses. They are known as cruciferous because their flowers are cross shaped. One cup of cooked broccoli provides half a day's supply of vitamin A in form of beta-carotene, twice the requirement of vitamin C, 9% of calcium, 12% of phosphorus, 10% of iron, 20% of daily fibre needs, some amount of protein, potassium, and 45 calories. One of these phytochemicals, sulforaphane plays a role in cancer prevention. Humans who eat large amounts of cruciferous vegetables are at lower risk of cancers. It is suspected that the combination of beta-carotene, in-doles and isothiocynates work together to offer this protection. Other members of the cruciferous family include: Cabbage, kale, Cauliflower and Brussels sprout which are high in nutritional value but not as much as broccoli.

PROTEINS AND DAIRY PRODUCTS
Proteins are macromolecules of amino acids. They form about 40% of dry weight of cells. This is why our body needs good quantity of proteins each day for growth, tissue repairs, maintenance of body mass and for manufacture of different enzymes and neurotransmitters. Proteins are obtained from both animal and plant sources. It is now known that vegetables can supply our daily protein needs.

Nuts, grains, seeds, green vegetables and soy products, legumes and potatoes with skin are good sources of protein which are easy to digest. They contain fibre.

Meat contains large quantities of saturated fats and cholesterol. Cholesterol hardens and narrows arteries leading to high blood pressure and other heart diseases. Every 30 seconds someone dies of heart diseases due to animal fat. Meat contains much uric acid which causes arthritis and gout. The uric acid can overstretch the kidneys while trying to excrete the uric acid. Meat has no dietary fibres which maintain good integrity of the gut and prevent chronic diseases and cancer. Meat creates an acidic environment preferred by cancer cells. It should be noted that carnivores (meat eating animals) have highly acidic stomach where the meat is easily digested.

Man did not eat animal as food until after the flood. This shortened his lifespan from 900 to 70 years.

LIST OF SOME VEGETABLES THAT ARE GOOD FOR HEALTH

BIOLOGY NAME	LOCAL COMMON NAME
Telferia occidentalis	Fluted pumkin (Ugu in igbo)
Amaranthus hybridus	Pigweed (inine in igbo, tete in yoruba)
Corcorus olitorius	Jute (ewedu in yoruba)
Gnetum bucholzianam	Koko vine (okazi in igbo, afang in ibibio)
Gongronema latifolium	Utazi (in igbo)
Heinsia crinite	Atama (Anang)
Pterocarpus mildbraedii	Oha (in igbo)
pterocarpus santalinoides	Red sandalwood, (nturukpa in igbo)
Salanum melongena	Egg plant, (afufa in igbo, igba in yoruba)
Talinum triangulare	Water leaf
Verononia amygdalina	Bitter leaf (Onugbu in igbo, ewuru in yoruba)

Man's
molar teeth are for grinding not for tearing as in carnivores. Our digestive system is typical of vegetarian diet. Meat is associated with risk of cancers because of carcinogens produced while going through our digestive system and are reabsorbed. One of the carcinogens of beef is benzopyrene. When prepared at high temperatures e.g. pan frying produces hetero-cyclic amine (HCA) which is a carcinogen. Therefore remove red meat from your diet.

Red meat increases risk of esophageal and stomach cancers (Am Journal of Gastroenterology N: 494979). Those who always eat red meat had 79% risk of developing upper esophageal and colon cancer.

Colon cancer risk

Frequency of eating beef, pork lamb		percentage increase
1	Less than one ounce	0
2	One ounce per month to one per week	39
3	Two to four times per week	50
4	Five to six time per week	84
5	Daily or more	149

Dr. Illmari and Kamerva reported a 67 percent drop in deaths due to heart diseases during I & II World wars because of the significant drop in meat, eggs, milk, butter, cheese and lard. The drop was due to disruption of the distribution of processed food during the wars.

Almost all foods except table sugar and pure fat contain some proteins.

We do not have good enzymes to digest meat which therefore putrefies during its long journey along the intestines. This putrefaction produces carcinogens which are reabsorbed into the body.

Plant proteins are associated with dietary fibres and constitute one of the most important elements of a healthy diet.

Fish is reach in Omega-3 fatty acids which reduce low density lipoprotein (LDL bad cholesterol) and triglycerides and increase good (HDL) cholesterol. Fish contains large quantities of potassium, iron, magnesium, zinc and vitamin A, B and D.

however sea foods such as shell fish, shrimps, cod, salmon, sardines, mackerels are preferred to fish.

MILK: While it is considered a complete and perfect food, recent researches have revealed startling findings on the bad side of milk.

It has been found that animal milk is best suited for the species that produces it. Because of this, the best milk for man is our mothers' breast milk.
Milk is most needed during infancy when the infant cannot eat another food.

This is why today scientists and nutritionists advocate mothers exclusively breast feeding their infants. It has been shown that the composition of breast milk suits our infants. Example, about 1.2% of breast milk is protein while cow milk contains 3.3%. This protein is made up of casein (curd protein) and whey proteins (lactalbumin and lactoglobulin). Cow milk contains six times more casein than breast milk. It should be noted that before most milk products reach our dining table their bioactivity is almost entirely lost although their food value remains. This is due to pasteurization and other industrial processes that cow milk undergoes, thus it is not useful especially for adults (M.K. Gupta. Foods that are killing you)
Recent studies now support that consumption of dairy milk products and sucrose (table sugar) is associated with higher risk of developing cancers especially colon, ovarian and breast cancers.
Proteins in milk are responsible for many cases of heart diseases. Milk has a lot of saturated fats that are risk factors for cancers. The poly-unsaturated fatty acids in milk could lead to cancer formation by generating free radicals.

While infants and young people have inbuilt systems that mop up free radicals, this system breaks down in adulthood, leaving us with high risks of developing cancers and other non-communicable diseases. Dairy   products   include   milk, cheese, ice creams, butter and cakes.

Prof Jane Plant, a breast cancer patient was cured of her disease through dairy regulations. With her cancer, she ate a lot of yoghurt to increase her probiotics to help her. She also had courses of chemotherapy with very little effects. When she boycotted all dairy products, her axillary and cervical lymphadenopathy (enlarged nodes) started to shrink. Within six weeks, she added an hour meditation. Her lymph nodes disappeared. When her doctors could not find the lymph nodes, she declared "I now believe that the link between dairy products and breast cancer is similar to the link between smoking and lung cancer". She also affirms that coloured fruits, vegetables "have the most potent punch on breast cancer" (Nig. Sat Punch 13/03/10). Every woman should examine her breast regularly because the chance of developing breast cancer in life is one in eight.

Dr. Day, an orthopedic surgeon for 25 years before she had breast cancer, refused surgery, radiation and chemotherapy. She was cured of her cancer by removing dairy products from her menu and depended completely on natural foods. In view of the above testimonies I advise staying away from dairy products.

SUGARS

Sugar belongs to a group of our daily foods called carbohydrates. The simplest form of carbohydrate is the monosaccharide, called simple sugars. Its formula is $C_6H_{12}O_6$. They include Glucose, fructose and galactose. Our table sugar belongs to the group of carbohydrates called disaccharides ($C_{12}H_{22}O_{11}$) because it is made up of two molecules of monosaccharide.

The most common disaccharide is cane sugar, called sucrose. It consists of one molecule of glucose and one molecule of fructose. We shall discuss this in greater detail here.

Lactose is the milk sugar and makes up half of the total solid in milk. It consists of glucose and galactose.

Maltose is the malt sugar. It consists of two molecules of glucose.

Polysaccharides are made up of many molecules of monosaccharide ($C_6H_{10}O_5$) n. It is found in starch, cellulose, dextrin and glycogen.

The disaccharides are digested to form simple sugars. All simple sugars are converted to glucose by the liver. Glucose is then oxidized to produce the energy required for carrying out body activities.

$$C_6H_{12}O_6 + 6O_2 \longrightarrow 6CO_2 + 6H_2O + Energy$$
glucose + Oxygen   Carbon dioxide + Water

Excess glucose is converted by the liver to glycogen which is stored in the liver and muscles. The brain burns 2/3 of body glucose which generates 20 to 25 watts of electricity needed to conduct the brain's electrical activities in 24hrs. The brain uses glucose exclusively as its source of energy. The brain is dependent on a minute to minute supply of this glucose because of its rapid metabolic rate of 7.5 times greater than the average body tissue. The brain accounts for 15 percent of our total metabolism. The best sources of carbohydrates for the brain are fruits, vegetables and whole grains. Animal products are almost devoid of carbohydrates. From the afore-going, sugar is very important in our lives. It is the quality and quantity of sugar we take that may produce harmful effects on us.

TABLE SUGARS: The table sugar we consume is a very unnatural chemical. It is a disaccharide; sucrose. Plant sugar from cane (or beet) plant is pressed and the juices collected. This juice is refined into molasses, then to brown sugar (or sucrose) and finally the strange white crystals $C_{12}H_{22}O_{11}$-Caramel, which is devoid of any fibres. During these refining processes at 180°C all the vitamins, minerals, proteins, enzymes and other beneficial nutrients in the cane (un-refined) sugar are destroyed. We are now left with a concentrated un-natural substance that the body cannot handle; at least in the quantities we consume it. Refined sugar is bad because:

1)   It has very little nutritional value

2)   It breaks down very quickly in the body leaving excess glucose floating around in the blood. This creates a panic situation, which results in the pancreas releasing a large quantity of insulin to compensate or remove the excess glucose by storing same as glycogen.

3)   The worst side of sugar is the damage it does on global health. Types 2 diabetes or non-insulin dependent diabetes is on the increase worldwide.

4)   It depletes B vitamins from body stores. Since these vitamins required for digestion and assimilation are lacking in sugar, the digestion and assimilation extract   the
vitamins from muscles, liver, kidney, heart and skin. If depletion continues, the resultant situation is nervous irritability, digestive disorders and cardiovascular diseases.

5)   Ten recent studies have linked sugar to increased cancer risks because cancer cells need significantly more glucose to grow and thrive than normal cells. They make use of it where normal cells cannot, by use of AKC protein.

6) The resultant out-pouring of insulin could result in a low sugar level in the blood called hypoglycemia which manifests as dizziness, tiredness, tremor and nausea.

To avoid this unhealthy rise and fall of blood sugar levels, we should start each day with high quantity breakfast that includes balanced plant sources.

7) Sugar causes tooth decay because the sugar particles which get stuck on gums are fermented to produce acids which erode the teeth.

8) Sugar increases acidity in the blood. (MK. Gupta: Foods that are killing you)

Good natural sources of sugar include:
1)   Sugarcane juice with its rich content of vitamins B & C and fibres.

2)   Fruit sugars are balanced with vitamins and fibres to slow down its digestion to glucose and subsequent panic increase in blood sugar (hyperglycemia). The fruits include: Oranges, grapes, banana, carrot, paw-paw, apples to name a few. The fruits should not be over-ripe.

3)   Honey contains 75 percent sugar but has numerous micronutrients required by a healthy body. Honey is alkaline and does not produce acidosis.

4)   Thaumatin: It is the sweetest natural product known to mankind. (Guardian 20/11/08)

Aspartame (NutraSweet). It is an artificial sweetener shown to cause breast cancer and leukemia in animal experiments. Sweeteners contain neither calories nor fibres. Aspartame is used in over 4000 processed products worldwide. It is said to be exo-cytotic because of the nerve cell damage caused by its breakdown products methyl alcohol and formaldehyde. It causes influx of calcium into brain cells triggering off excessive amounts of free radicals which damage the cells. Some of these effects include macular degeneration and retinopathy (disease of the eye) now seen more in younger age groups and may cause blindness. Claims that these by-products are detoxified by the liver may be true but for how long will the liver do this without breaking down. (Guardian 20/11/08)

Formaldehyde accumulates near DNA and causes serious damage interfering with its replication. Consistent ingestion of processed foods by people with risk factors for Diabetes mellitus and cancer places them at a higher risk for these diseases. However, large volumes of scientific evidences show link between aspartame, sugar and increased cancer risk.

There are clear associations between high glycemic index foods and colorectal cancers. These foods include candy bars, cakes, cookies and other snacks. These glycemic foods give 135 percent higher risk for breast cancer in 7 years (n= 40,000. Women), 46 percent for pancreatic cancers (n=90,000-USA women), 57 percent higher risk for prostate cancers. (USA Nurses HL study for 18yrs)

We should avoid simple sugars and sweeteners in processed and refined foods, including soft drinks, sugary beverages, candy bars, cakes etc. These cause our insulin levels to spike because of hyperglycemia (high blood sugar). Sugar triggers chronic inflammations which disrupt the immune system which results to havoc in the brain and cause heart diseases, Diabetes, Arthritis and cancer. A combination of sugar and milk will likely cause fermentation in the stomach and are thus harmful. Sugar when largely used is more injurious than meat.

Other Food Sweeteners and Chemicals:
Other food additive substances are added to our foods to enhance textures, enriching food values e.g. with Vitamins and mineral. The most ancient additive is sodium chloride (Table salt). The use of red pepper in Nigeria is prehistoric.

It is estimated that 10,000 additives find their way into food processing and packages, including unwanted ones like pesticides used to preserve seeds and fruits.

While producers of these products claim they are safe their interactions with other chemicals and the cumulative effects are still controversial. For example, the nitrates added to meat to preserve its colour, reacts with amino acids in the stomach to produce carcinogenic nitrosamines.
Aspartame and saccharin; artificial sweeteners, that have been used over many years, are now banned in developed countries because of their effects on human life.

Monosodium glutamate (MSG) - Chinese salt: It is one of the best flavor enhancers. It is also banned in many countries because it damages brain cells and causes kidney failure. In Nigeria, National Agency for Food and Drugs Administration and Control (NAFDAC) is at war with bakers who add it to enhance bread. It is because of these known and unknown information about additives that we are advised to return to natural foods.

The high level of sugars in soft drinks causes increased insulin production by pancreatic cells predisposing one to pancreatic cancer. Though rare, pancreatic cancer is one of the most deadly cancers.

TABLE SALT/COMMON SALT

The chemical name of common salt is sodium chloride (NaCl). Sodium hardly occurs free in nature. Common salt is obtained from sea water and land deposits. It is one of the oldest food additives known to man. The body needs about ½ teaspoonful of salt daily. This should be less in families with history of hypertension. The blood content of sodium compared to other elements is as follows.

Na 137-144 mmol/litre, potassium 3.5-4.8, calcium 2.12-2.62, magnesium 0.7-1.0, copper 13-24, all measurements are in mmol.

This underscores its importance to us. We should take sun dried salt and not oven/kiln dried salt. Like sugar, all minerals, about 80 of them, and vitamins are destroyed during the refining processes. Food additives are used to give it its bright colour and reduce clumps. These additives are carcinogenic.

Functions of salt in the body:

(1)   Water, salt and potassium together regulate the water content of the body.

(2)   There are two oceans of water in the body, one held inside the cell; Intracellular and the other outside-extracellular, in interstitial spaces, lymph and blood. The volumes of these oceans are maintained by the mineral content of natural salt. Good health could be measured, by the balance between the two volumes of water and its mineral content.

(3)   Salt helps because its mineral content makes the inside of cells alkaline which is essential for prevention and treatment of cancers.

(4)   We need salt to expand the blood volume so that it stays dilute and reaches all nooks and crannies of the body.

(5)   It is an important constituent of blood (0.9gm/100ml).

(6)	It helps in conduction of impulses. It is a key factor in the electrical activities of the heart.

(7)	It helps transport substances across cell membranes.

(8)	The chloride content helps to produces HCl in the stomach.

(9)	Sodium helps maintain acid base balance in body fluids; blood, lymph, tears and gastro-intestinal secretions.

Excessive intake causes:

(1)	Increased blood pressure by water retention.

(2)	Imposes great burden on the kidneys which try to excrete the excess.

(3)	Worsens edema.

(4)	Increases uric acid in the body thus worsening uric acid related illness, like gout.

It is important to note that most fruits, nuts, cereals contain good quantities of sodium where it is loosely bonded and easily available for body mechanisms. On the other hand many processed foods contain high quantities of salt e.g. cornflakes, potato and plantain chips, salted biscuits, fast foods and drinks to name a few. We should therefore be careful in choice of these foods.

It is therefore advisable that we consume moderate amounts of table salt preferably unprocessed rock salts which still retain most of its other minerals.

TOBACCO AND SMOKING

The active ingredient in tobacco is nicotine which gives the consumer a temporary lift by stimulating the pleasure centre thus making him feel high. He soon craves for more.

Tobacco is consumed as:

(1)	Cigarette and

(2)	Cigar, which are smoked.

(3)   Other forms include chewing tobacco leaves, sniffing ground tobacco leaves powder and mouth gargling with ground tobacco.

(4)   In USA current smokers, 60-90%, began at 14-19 years of age.

Actions of Tobacco in the Body

A puff of cigarette releases trillions of free radicals which cause inflammation in the tissues. This inflammation is the principal source of oxidative stress in humans. Nicotine in a puff reaches the brain in 6-8 seconds where it stimulates release of neurotransmitters. All its carcinogens gain easy access to the lung tissue. It is the worst risk factor for chronic obstructive pulmonary disease (COPD) and lung cancer. Higher doses stimulate the release of adrenaline and nor-adrenaline.

Diseases due to Smoking Tobacco

Tobacco is linked to 15 different cancers of the respiratory tract. Smoking related cancers account for 40 percent of cancer deaths in men, 5 times more in men than women. Smoking tobacco accounts for 85 percent of primary lung cancers.

There are about 599 approved additives in a stick of cigarette and its smoke is proven to contain over 4000 toxic carcinogens (cancer causing chemicals). These include carbon monoxide, nitrogen oxide, hydrogen cyanide, tar and ammonia, to name a few.

Low pricing, high status attached to smoking and exceptive advertisements have lured about 14 percent of Nigerians into smoking of which about 7 percent will die of tobacco related ailments.

The carcinogens in cigarette cause cancers of the lungs, throat, mouth, esophagus (gullet) and bladder. Smoking is a serious risk factor for most cardiovascular diseases.

Tobacco damages sperm cells making them less likely to fertilize eggs (Human Rep 07/09/10/Nig. Guardian 16/09/10)
It increases the rate of abortions, sudden fetal deaths and low birth weight babies.

It causes or worsens diabetes since it causes production of adrenaline and noradrenaline which push up blood sugar.

Statistics on Hazards of Smoking
About 1 in 3 cancer deaths is due to smoking.
About 1 in 5 deaths from cardiac disease is due to smoking.
About 9 out of 10 deaths from bronchitis, emphysema
Other chronic obstructive pulmonary diseases (COPD) are due to smoking.
An average smoker loses 8 years of his life to cigarette. Smokers have 70 percent overall death rates compared to non-smokers.
Risk of coronary heart disease is double in smokers compared to non-smokers.
Sudden death is 4 times more in young smokers than in non-smokers.
500 million people living today will ultimately die as a result of cigarette smoking.
World Health Organization (WHO) estimates that smoking causes 3 million deaths per year worldwide.
Tobacco users be warned.

ALCOHOL

Alcohol is also known to the scientist as ethanol or ethyl alcohol (ethanol CH_3CH_2OH)

For cancer prevention, it is best not to drink alcohol.

One in 25 deaths worldwide is directly linked to alcohol consumption. Most disabling diseases especially in elderly men are attributed to alcohol but its greatest burden lies with younger people. Most of the deaths caused by alcohol are through injuries, cancers, cardiovascular diseases and liver cirrhosis. The burden of alcohol nearly equals that of smoking especially in the most populous countries in developing economies, in India and China.

These effects of alcohol result in the following diseases:
1. Dementia.
2. Liver Cirrhosis.
3. Primary liver cell carcinoma.
4. Chronic hepatitis.
5. Polyneuritis.
6. Evidences abound that heavy consumption of alcohol increases the risk of developing prostate cancer.
7. Benign tremors are aggravated by chronic alcohol consumption as can be seen when holding up a cup by an alcoholic.
8. Alcoholism causes mal-absorption due to pancreatic and small bowel damage.
9 .Excessive drinking of alcohol causes peptic ulcer.
10 .Deficiencies of the B Vitamins and thiamine thus aggravating diseases that depend on these vitamins by causing alcoholic neuropathy.
11 .Mental and moral debility, unnatural appetite and highly irritable individuals.

12. Alcohol dependence. The suffering of his neighbors may be extraordinary. The consequences of alcohol abuse include spouse abuse, child abuse, neglect, suicide and industrial accidents and road traffic accidents (RTA).
13. Decreases ability to think abstractly and to make best moral decisions.

HOW ALCOHOL AFFECTS THE BODY
1 .It depletes the minerals and vitamins, and other immune boosting substances in the body thus suppressing the immune system, predisposing the victim to chronic and debilitating diseases including cancers.
2. Its diuretic effects on the liver and kidneys are unquantifiable.
3. It produces free radicals (Oxy-radicals), which attack and damage sensitive tissues causing many diseases in the body.
4. It produces brain dehydration which presents as hangover headache.
5. It causes a "Never-look-well" on its victims as seen in severe alcoholics.
6. Excessive consumption of alcohol leads to accumulation of the reduced form of Nicotinamide Adenine dinucleotide (NADH) which inhibits gluconeogenesis by preventing the oxidation of lactate to pyruvate, thus reducing the energy that should have been released.

Ethanol alters the communications in brain cells. It should not be mentioned among us.

Some of the alcoholic beverages include: Beer, Wine, Whisky, Brandy, Rum and Gin.
Alcoholism is commonly associated with chronic smoking thus causing artificial increase in dopamine. No wonder the personality loss of alcoholics.

These two substances of abuse have synergistic effects creating more harm than their individual effects. Addiction to alcohol and other drugs causes serious vitamin, mineral, protein and enzyme deficiencies many of which are irreversible.

Ethanol cannot be excreted but must be metabolized by the liver using two pathways. Each of these pathways produces NADH (as shown above). Pathological consequences of alcohol consumption include:
The 1st stage - fatty liver.
The second stage: cirrhosis results.
Here, fibrous tissues and scar tissues are formed around cells. The biochemical functions of the liver are impaired e.g., ammonia, which is toxic, cannot be converted to urea which is excreted. This may cause coma and death. 75 percent of liver cirrhosis is as a result of alcoholism.

CAFFEINE

The coffee shrub was discovered in China thousands of years ago. Shepherds in the Arabian sub-continent who fed their goats with coffee discovered they climbed trees and ate anything they could chew, including roots. Caffeine is naturally found in kola nuts, coffee and tea.

It is found in chocolate, carbonated beverages energy drinks, cola and in some over-the counter medications. Many are easily identified by their coffee colour. Recent studies indicate that chronic consumption of caffeine containing beverages predisposes one to coronary heart diseases and glaucoma.

EFFECTS OF CAFFEINE ON THE BODY

Caffeine inhibits the action of phosphodiesterase enzymes in the nerve cells. This enzyme is pivotal in the process of memory formation and retention. It blocks the action of adenosine which has a calming effect on the nerves. Thus its stimulant effect is accentuated. The consumers crave for more: addiction. It stimulates the adrenal glands to produce stress hormones adrenaline, nor-adrenaline and cortisol, thus increasing stress levels. These actions are worse on the nerve cells in the brain. Smoking and alcohol reduce the half-life of coffee, thus smokers and alcoholics can take more resulting in addiction.

Caffeine intoxication is characterized by:
Marked nervousness, anxiety, restlessness, insomnia (lack of sleep), tremors, rapid heartbeats (tachycardia) and, in rare cases death.
Many beverages contain coffee as mentioned above.
Caffeine is a diuretic (increases urine output) creating dehydration. This is why we get thirstier as we take cola drinks.
It has addictive properties because of its stimulating effects on nervous system and cardiac muscles.
It increases endurance in athletes. Caffeine draws up reserved energy especially in the brain cells resulting in hyperactivity even when we are tired. These energy stock piles are used up even when not necessary. This drawing up from energy reserves of cells frequently is the root cause of many health problems in caffeine consuming people.

This is what causes Attention Deficit Hyperactivity Disorder (ADHA) seen in children who take a lot of caffeinated beverages. There is increased intraocular pressure in high coffee consuming people.
In Nigeria accounts for 5% of heart attacks (Lancet 24/02/11)

High coffee consumers have a great tendency to hallucinate.
Coffee in pregnancy is associated with low birth weight.

Withdrawal symptoms include: Headache, fatigue, feeling less alert, less energetic and difficulty in concentration. It is therefore advisable that we remove coffee, kola nuts and caffeine beverages from our meals.

·"Alcohol adds another level of danger to coffee consumers because its high doses give false sense of alertness that provides incentive to drive a car thus putting themselves, their passengers and other road users in great danger" Griffiths.

Athletes who ingest caffeine and carbohydrates have glycogen (in muscles) replenished faster than in nonusers. As much as 66 percent more glycogen is seen in users' muscles 4 hours after exercise. This improves athlete performance.

Coffee and tea considerably lower the risk of type 2 diabetes or Non-insulin dependent diabetes.

WATER

The evolutionists make us understand that life started from water. This is why all forms of life depend on it for survival. The other elements of life are air and food. The importance of water to life is based on the fact that all physiological activities of the body depend on water. Therefore dehydration (shortage of water) of any degree in the body is bound to produce unquantifiable adverse effects on the body of any animal including humans. The elasticity of living organisms enables them make adjustments to survive under any harsh condition like dehydration. It is the failure of these adjustments to return the body to its former normal situation that produces most non-communicable diseases. From age of 20 we start suppressing our thirst and by age 45 the consequences are non-communicable diseases and cancers. Dr. F. Batmanghelidj's study of the importance of water in the body has not been equaled. I can only mention some of them to underscore the importance of water in our body. (F. Batmanghelidj's: Obesity, cancer, depression)

- It is water that enables hydrolysis to take place. It is a source of energy, even more than food. During hydrolysis, there is transfer of energy from water to the substrate being hydrolyzed.

Water is responsible for the manufacture of hydroelectricity for the functions of the brain.

- Certain proteins are found on the cell membranes. These proteins have affinity with certain minerals in the blood and interstitial fluids, around the cells. These minerals get attached to their specific proteins and are transported across cell membranes by the rush of water in and out of the cells. This process produces electricity that is stored in the form of ATP and GTP (Adenosine and Guanidine Triphosphate respectively).
- In dehydration; 66 percent of the water is lost from the interior of the cells, 26 percent loss is from the intracellular space and 8 percent is borne by the blood in the vascular system, which .constricts to maintain the integrity of the circulatory system.
- The brain is the most vulnerable organ which suffers the consequences of this dehydration.
- There are nine trillion brain and nerve cells in the body which constantly communicate with each other. This complicated activity is powered by hydroelectricity. This is why a glass of water is the best "pick-me-up drink". It will energize the brain and the entire body within minutes without waste materials.

- The human brain is about 1/50 of the total body weight. The brain cells are 85 percent water. About 20 percent of blood in circulation is made available to the brain per unit time. We can therefore imagine the effect of dehydration which offsets this balance.
- The brain expends a vast quantity of energy to process all information from the body and exposure to its physical, social and electromagnetic environments. It also expends lots of energy to manufacture the neurotransmitters and their transportation into nerve endings. Water transports all chemicals needed by the brain to manufacture its chemicals.
- Prevents DNA damage and makes its repair mechanisms more efficient.
- Increases the rate of absorption of essential substances in food into the body.
- Increases the efficiency of red blood cells in collecting oxygen in the lungs.
- Clears toxic wastes from different parts of the body to the liver, kidney and skin for excretion.
- Is the best laxative and prevents constipation.
- Is needed for the production of all hormones.
- Is vital for efficient immune system functions. About 1/6 of the human body is made up of interstitial spaces. This is filled with fluid lymph, which carries wastes away. Lymph is water with defense agents, macrophages, lymphocytes at the lymph nodes.
- Toxic sediments deposited in tissue spaces, fat stores, joints, kidneys, liver, brain and skin are cleared by water.
- Takes away morning sickness of pregnancy.

Consequences of dehydration

Kidneys (and lungs) regulate the acid and alkaline states of the body provided they receive enough water to produce good quantity of urine. The interior of cells maintain an alkaline state of about 7.4. In dehydration, the intracellular fluid becomes acidic. Together with toxins and free radicals at the intracellular spaces, the internal environments are altered. This causes alteration in the delicate structures of the cell including DNA. This damage is repaired when the cells are rehydrated. When destruction of DNA outstrips repair of DNA, transformations occur. The replication of these deformed DNA produces erratic cancer cells.

Dehydration· creates drought management situations with increased histamine production. Histamine stimulates prostaglandin production and subsequent pains as seen in low back pains, angina (pains from heart) and peptic ulcer. These are indicators of thirst and dehydration. A cup of water given to exacerbated peptic ulcer pains gives remarkable relieve within 30 minutes to the patient.

In dehydration, the adrenal glands release a lot of hormones, including cortisol, cortisone and aldosterone. Cortisol and cortisone are strong anti-inflammatory agents, consequently suppressing the immune system. This situation further aggravates cancer formations.

Regimen and Doses of water

An average weight person (60kg) requires about 4.5 litres of water daily, 2.5 litres is "free water" while 2 litres come from metabolism and food water content. Free water here refers to water taken when the stomach is empty of food to enable the body absorb it completely. It also replenishes water lost through urine, perspiration and breathing. Normal urine output is 1.5 - 2 litres daily and even less in the tropics and in the heavily built. The free water enables us to attain this urine output, rehydrates cells and produces a fast flowing 'stream' in our body that washes away wastes.

Take at least one litre first thing in the morning.

This replaces water lost during the night.

It enables you to produce enough urine to clean your body of wastes toxins, free radicals, urine produced during metabolism at night. It softens the stool to enable you empty the toxic wastes in faces almost completely.

It is advisable to repeat the volume of free water at least 1 hour before lunch and dinner. This free water is also termed "Therapeutic water" because of the afore-mentioned uses of the water.

Take at least a glass of water; 10 minutes before a meal. This prepares the enzymes ready for the digestion of the incoming food.

Before any exercise drink a lot of water, because much water is lost during exercise. The water also helps eliminate wastes produced during exercise.

The water you drink with food is "bound water" because it is used for digestion and is not free for immediate absorption.

Water before meals prevents gastro-intestinal tract problems - bloating, heartburn, colitis, constipation, cancers of the intestinal tract and weight gain.

Drink at regular interval to avoid dehydration.

A little bit of unrefined salt, from soil or sea will provide a lot of minerals needed by the body.

MINERALS

POTASSIUM

It is the principal regulator of intracellular water. As it gets into the cell it pulls a large quantity of water thus ensuring that the cell is well hydrated. The sodium-potassium exchange pump ensures adequate distribution of these elements inside and outside the   cell.

Foods with high potassium content include oranges, potatoes, avocado peas, banana, tomatoes, whole wheat bread and eggs.

SELENIUM:

Selenium is mostly required for the functioning of the immune system. 'Though required in small quantities, its shortages results in low levels of the enzyme glutathione peroxidase seen in many cancer patients. Its effects as an antioxidant are discussed elsewhere in this book. Its sources include: different nuts, wheat germ, whole wheat, brown rice, shrimps, mushrooms, garlic, oranges, fish, and cooked chickens.

MAGNESIUM:

It is the element that gives stability to all energy dependent processes in the body. It is the source of the energy that facilitates the fine but complex communications between the nine trillion brain nerve cells. It plays a very vital role in the life span of cells, thus lack of it results in reduced efficiency of cells. It is involved in more than 300 enzymatic reactions in the metabolism of food substances.

Since hard water is a source of magnesium, those who drink it are less prone to heart diseases. Its deficiency worsens hypertension and irregular heartbeats (arrhythmia). Carbonated drinks and sodas contain much phosphate which depletes magnesium in the body. It plays very important role in proper functioning of the immune system and in recovery from illnesses, including cancers.

Its main sources are: Green chlorophyll in vegetables, fruits, and seeds, peas, wheat bran, nut, peanuts, brown rice, avocado pears, milk and eggs.

CALCIUM
Calcium is the most abundant mineral in the body. It is held tenaciously in the bones where it forms the bulk of its weight. Its deficiency therefore causes weakening of bones - osteoporosis which predisposes the bones to easy fracture. The direct consequence of dehydration is formation of kidney stones. This is why the best treatment for and prevention of kidney stones is intake of good quantity of water.

All organs that secrete hormones and manufacture enzymes for digestion depend on calcium for release of their products.

Magnesium and calcium pump also produces energy for the cells as the sodium potassium pumps.

Its sources include beans, pumpkin seeds, nuts, dried fruits, egg, milk, sesame seeds, potatoes and all green vegetables.

VITAMIN E
Vitamin E interferes with the ability of prostate cells to make both prostate specific antigen (PSA) and androgen receptors. These are key players in development and progression of prostate cancer. Vitamin E succinate (alphatophenyl succinate) is the most effective form.(USA NAS 28/05.03)

Vitamin E Succinate works by blocking a protein called Bcl-xl. This protein is made by healthy cells and often found in abnormally high levels in cancer cells and protect them from dying when they should. Its antioxidant effects are well known to science today.

Beverage	Percentage alcohol
Beer	3-8%
Wine	10-20%
Whisky	50%
Brandy	56 -60%
Rum	40%
Gin	40%

(M.K Gupta. Foods that are killing you)

CHAPTER FOUR

BALANCED DIET

A balanced diet consists of very little animal proteins and animal fat, water, little carbohydrate and lots of natural plant products. Beans, grains contain 25 percent proteins, Vegetables contain 15 percent proteins. Fruits have good vegetable sugar. We should aim at eating 65-75% of our food raw because of the antioxidants content. The body needs fruits and vegetables daily as they are sources of natural vitamins and minerals that we need.

OUR MENU

Breakfast should be heavier than other meals of the day:

At this time the stomach is empty and can accommodate more food.

Since we are more active during the morning hours, more food will supply the much needed energy to cope with the stress of our daily activities.

It will reduce the risk of stress ulcers.

Those working on their weights should note that heavy dinner is followed by a long period of inactivity. This quantity of food is stored thus increasing weights.

Late night meals are not good because. They are not digested before bedtime.

The digestive system does not have proper rest.

Sleep is disturbed.

The brain and nerves are over worked, when they should be resting.

Appetite for breakfast is impaired.

The whole digestive system is un-refreshed and not ready for the next day's activities.

Where a third meal may .be required, according to individual Circumstances, it should be very light. As much as possible, meals should be at regular times.

Breakfast: High quality breakfast should include a balanced choice of plant foods.
1)   Soya bean powder drink.
2)   Soya milk.
3)   Raw fruits e.g. tomatoes, mangoes, pumpkin fruit, lettuce, cabbage.
4)   Avocado peas
5)   Whole wheat bread
6)   Onions, garlic, ginger.
7)   Beans, garri, okpa (Igbo)

Mid-morning (Tea) break
1)   Fruits
2)   Homemade fruit juices from carrots, paw-paw.
3)   Walnuts.
4)   Water.

Lunch
1)   Fruits "Ukwa" – (Igbo).
2)   Plenty vegetables.
3)   Carbohydrates - Yam, garri, unpolished rice, beans.

Evening (Tea) break
1)   Fruits.
2)   Homemade juices
3)   Walnuts, "Ukwa" - Igbo.
4)   Water.

Dinner
1)   Very small quantities of unpolished rice, potatoes, beans.
2)   Plenty vegetables.
Freshly prepared homemade juices of carrot, water melon, pineapples, plant leaves, bitter leaves, cabbage, enrich our menu but are better taken "empty" stomach so that much of the nutrients they contain can be freely absorbed. Today, those who are purely vegetarians (Gen 1:29) as directed by God live healthier longer lives with much fewer chronic non communicable diseases.

Adequate and timely intake of water as discussed elsewhere in this book completes our menu.

Good quantity of water taken 10 minutes before meals reduces our food intake. This aids weight loss.

CONCLUSION

THE ARK OF NOAH. Many asked what he was doing when he was building the boat. He was not deterred by people's comments. At the end, he alone and his household survived the flood. This little book may be reminding us that we do not have to wait for the 'flood' before we start building our boat for the rains. Every one of us is at risk. By the time we are 45-50 years and above, one of the non-communicable diseases or cancer is lurking through the "crack on our walls". YES we must die of an ailment but we can add a few more years of active useful life to ourselves, by change of lifestyle, diet and exercise.

While this book is not a treatise on diet and longevity, the contents are worth living out. You may be one of the "spontaneously" healed because in scientific trials there are some among the control groups who do as well as those on the trials, God is ALIVE and he chooses those He will favour anytime.

In science, the final truth is always, somewhere beyond our grasp.

It is for this reason that the barrier between conventional medicine and complementary medicine should be broken so that they call for a dialogue since the truth lies beyond the grasp of both practitioners. It is gratifying to note that some primary care centres and hospitals in Britain now offer complementary medicine as well as conventional medicines. Let us learn from them.

While complementary practitioners claim that their products are natural and thus non- toxic, producers of orthodox drugs do agree that many of their products are toxic and do not work. "The vast majority of our drugs, more than 90 percent, only work in 30 or 50 percent of the people (British Independent 08/12/03, Glaxo Chief: our drugs do not work on most patients).

Annually, 2 million Americans become seriously ill from drug toxicity to correctly prescribed drugs taken properly and 106,000 die from these drug reactions, making drugs side effects the sixth most common cause of death in USA (The Washington post, 15/04/98).

Elements of cancer protective lifestyle are recommended for all and sundry.

1.   Proper diet with high fibre from
        ·   Fruits.
        ·   Vegetables - dark green, deep yellow, red
        ·   Cereals and grains.
        ·   Nuts.
2.   Maintain proper body weight. BMI <30. Do not dig your graves with knives and forks, overfed   yet malnourished.
3.   Regular meals with no snacks.
4.   Regular aerobic exercises; 30 mins, 5 times weekly or H.I.T daily
5.   Sunlight in moderation.
6.   Stress control.
7.   Do not smoke.
8.   7 -8 hours of sleep every night.
9.   Refrain from alcohol.
10.   Enjoy a hearty and well balanced breakfast.
11.   Know your numbers normal ranges
        Blood pressure
        Blood sugar
        Cholesterol
12.   Drinking plenty water; not less than 2.5 liters/day

People aged 45 and above who practice six of these health habits would normally live 33 more years. These health habits will definitely make a positive impact on the quality and longevity of your life.

The eight golden-laws of health will keep you alive even more healthy and longer. The eight remedies include: Pure water, fresh air, rest, temperance, sunlight, exercise, nutrition and trust in God, all already discussed.

May I end this book with the pleasant song that reminds us that our God is good.

You are the Lord that healeth me
You are the Lord my healer
You sent your word and healed my disease
You are the Lord my healer. (Repeat)

MEDICAL TIT BITS

1) The global battle today is for the preservation of our freedom to vitamins, minerals, proteins and all other natural therapies. (Dr. Rath led breakthrough on vitamins and cardiovascular diseases).
2) Today the most common diseases are recognized to be the direct result of nutrition deficiencies.
Therefore virtually all these disease are preventable in many natural ways.
3) The pharmaceutical industry has created the fourth largest epidemic that haunts mankind, the drug side effect epidemic (JAMA< April 15, 1998)
4) All cholesterol-lowering drugs currently in the market cause cancer and should be avoided (JAMA06/01 /96)
5) It is now superstitious to even think that any of us can get all the nutrients for optimum health from dietary nutrition alone.
6) Over half of US population now seek alternative to orthodox medicine (Dr. Weill)
7) The body's internal soldiers consist largely of the immune system, with its NK, -or natural killer Cell Defense. The WBCs .are always alert to search and destroy invaders completely.

8) Additions to alcohol and drugs cause serious vitamin, mineral, protein and enzyme deficiencies that manifest as devastating neurological diseases, many of which are irreversible.

9) Vitamins function as Co-enzymes.

10) The body's immune system weighs about 2.2pounds (1kg). The immune system performs the following functions (1)Recognizes invaders (2).Reacts to each invader (3)1t must remember and repel similar invasions by using hormone-like signal substances called transfer factors. These factors are made up of small peptides of amino acid residues that can be combined to make billions of different factors.

Some Health Commandments:

1)   Thou shall abstain from all unnatural, de-vitaminized food and stimulating beverages.

2)   Thou shall nourish the body with only natural, unprocessed live foods.

3)   Thou shall keep thy thoughts, words and emotions, pure, calm and uplifting.

Science has identified 13 modern day lifestyles that are increasing the risk of premature deaths.

Sitting for long hours of work

Watching too much TV

Heavy coffee consumption

Remaining unmarried

Early retirement

Prolonged air pollution

Taking afternoon nap

Constantly arguing

Poor dental hygiene/not brushing the teeth

Abuse of common pain killers

Heavy smoking and drinking
Growing patronage of processed food/red meat
Sugary drinks
(By world health statistics 2014)

13 FOODS THAT MAKE YOU AGE FAST
Fast foods
Processed meat
High salt meal-make you 10 years older, dehydrate you, and give high Blood pressure
Coffee, a high level of caffeine dehydrates you
Alcohol-liver disease, fatty liver, wrinkled skin
Energy drinks-destroy your teeth, high level of caffeine and taurine-HCL
Mineral (soft drinks)
White sugar-has no health benefit. It increases cholesterol, provides empty calorie and causes diabetes mellitus (DM), fatty liver and cancer.
Artificial sweeteners-saccharine, Aspartame, cause joint pains headache, rapid aging.
Microwave foods-cause water retention and contain excess Sodium
Red meat especially cow meat-fatty meat, cow moving poisons, cholesterol.
  Spicy foods
Lemonade/lemon juices
Carbohydrate only diets

14 FOODS TO AVOID AFTER A WORK OUT-SPORTS, GYM, FRAMEWORK, SERIOUS PRAYER SESSIONS, FASTING.

1. 1Raw vegetables-utazi, ukazi ,bitter leaf, bitter kola-leads to drop in BP and blood sugar
2. Fried foods
3. Crisps e g. potato, plantain-contains too much salt so leads to potassium loss
4. Shawarma (pizza) meat pie
5. Fizzy/soft drinks-drink water when you are thirsty or milk or yoghurt, they contain much sugar/chemical
6. Chocolate-too much sugar and empty calories
7. Energy/candy bars needed before exercise and not after because of high calories.
8. Energy drinks-needed before workout
9. Spicy foods-heartburn and indigestion
10. Abbacha (cassava peelings)-contain fibres but poor calories
11. Avocado-high in fats, best 2 hours before and 2 hours after work out
12. Granular bars
13. Cheese/cakes-processed fats
14. Processed meat-ham salami bacon

Drink-water, eat a balanced diet

-Banana

-Apple

-Water melon

-Chicken

-Fish

5 FOODS THAT ARE DISTROYING YOUR TEETH

1. Dried fruit- e.g date (debino)
2. Chewable vitamins
3. Barbecue sauce

4. Juice-use straw, wait for 40 minutes before washing your teeth.
5. Wine (red & white) –contains acids that soften your teeth enamel.

5 SINFUL FOODS & SNACKS TO AVIOD AT ALL COSTS

1. Cheese balls
2. Sweets/soft cheese

3. Popcorn-much fat, sugar. Polythene package contains PFVA: (perfluorooctanoic acid) a cancerous chemical
4. Diet, soft drinks, contain zero calories but loaded with chemical colors and artificial sweeteners.
5. Canned foods- contain heavy amounts of sugar and chemicals added to increase shell life.

GOOD REASONS WHY A LARGE BREAKFAST IS HEALTHY

1. Boosts metabolism
2. Stabilizes your weight
3. Helps maintain a healthy diet

(Worst breakfast foods are sweet corn flakes, drinks etc.)

4. Increases concentration and help you stay focused and alert
5. Improves your mood
6. You burn much carbohydrates because it's the food of your most active period of the day

6 TOXIC FOODS THAT PEOPLE CONSUME ON A REGULAR BASIS

1. Almonds – wild almond contain cyanlde-tolal poison
2. Tomato stems-contain tuornatin-a poisonous substance used as pesticide
3. Raw honey-risk botulism, a neurotoxin

4. Cherry seeds –contain pirs, amygdalin- a toxic substances
5. Eggs –contains salmonella, cook it properly, avoid raw eggs or half done
6. Oysters and raw fish-- contain vibrio vulnificus- a very toxic germ

5 FOODS YOU SHOULD AVOID
1. Salad cream
2. white sugar
3. white bread
4. Fried food
5. White rice

23 FAT FIGHTING FOODS
1. Yoghurt
2. Guinea corn
3. Cinnamon (scent leaf-nchuanwu))
4. Hot peppers
5. Green tea
6. Grape fruits
7. Water melon
8. Peas and apples
9. Berries
10. Raw vegetables
11. Sweet potatoes
12. Egg-has 75 calories for 7g of protein
13. Coffee
14. Quaker oat
15. Crisp bread
16. Chicken
17. Fish pepper soup
18. Salad without cream
19. Vinegar

20. Nuts
21. Plain popcorn put in a plate
22. Fish
23. Beans

UNHEALTHY FOODS THAT ARE WRONGLY CALLED HEALTHY FOODS

1. Plantain chips
2. Low fat yoghurt
3. Sport drinks-contains dyes, much sugar, chemicals
4. Can juice
5. Frozen foods

9 THINGS YOU SHOULD NEVER EAT OR DRINK AFTER 9.00PM

1. Milk especially adults
2. Pasta (macaroni, noddle)
3. Chocolate
4. Pizza
5. Pepper
6. Plenty of meat
7. Ginger/Chinese foods
8. suya
9. fruit juice-orange etc. cause heart burn

5 NIGERIAN FOODS TO AVOID LATE AT NIGHT

1. Amala and Ewedu
2. Pepper soup
3. Agege bread
4. Fried yam,akara,potatoes
5. Beans porridge with palm oil and pepper

NIGERIANS EAT POISON AS FOOD

- Moi moi and okpa wrapped in cellophane
- Pure water exposed to 28°C

- Cow meat contains TB
- Frozen chicken (preserved with formalin)
- Beans and grains preserved with pesticides

9 REASONS WHY YOU SHOULD GO TO BED ON EMPTY STOMACH (NOT EAT AFTER 8.00PM)

1. To avoid glucose spike at midnight and symptoms – drums, sweating.
2. To avoid overweight/obesity because sugars digested are not used so stored as fat.
3. To ensure good sleep (rapid eye movement sleep, rem)
4. To prevent gastritis, acid reflux
5. To prevent bad dreams
6. To enhance intake of breakfast
7. To lessen the risk of diabetes mellitus from pancreatic over work
8. To help prevent high blood pressure
9. To prevent lethargy, low mind, nervousness, blotted stomach at dawn

NOTE THIS RULE

Eat breakfast like a consultant (big man)
Lunch like a house officer (new doctor just managing to start life)
Dinner like a pediatric patient (a sick child hardly eats)

10 FOODS THAT MAKE YOU LOOK YOUNGER

1. morning coffee
2. Water melon
3. Pomegranates
4. Blue berries
5. Lobster
6. Leafy green vegetables
7. Eggs

8. Walnuts
9. Avocado pea
10. Water melon

REFERENCES

(1)   Batmanghelidj, Obesity, Cancer, Depression. Their common cause and natural cure, 2004.
(2)   Batmanghelidj: Your body's many cries for water.
(3)   Day, Lorraine. D.V.D. Cancer doesn't scare me anymore.
(4)   Ferrell, Vance: International meat crisis.
(5)   Guardian Newspaper. Natural Health review By: Emmanuel Muanya.
(6)   Guardian Newspaper: Science Guardian Review.
(7)   Gupta, M.K: Foods that are killing you slowly and steadily.
(8)   Gutman, Jimmy: GSH Your Body's most powerful protector Glutathione.
(9)   Nedley, Neil: Pray Positive.
(10)   Pfeifer, Ben L--Successful Natural Treatments for Breast and Prostate Cancers.
(11)   Lecture at complementary and Natural Healthcare Expo at Excel London on 15th October 2006.